Nursing Care Planning Guides

Set 4

Second Edition

SCHOOL OF PRACTICAL NURSING
LOUDOUN COUNTY SCHOOL BOARD
30 WEST NORTH STREET
LEESBURG, VIRGINIA 22075

AF711195

Nursing Care Planning Guides

Set 4

Second Edition

Margo Creighton Neal, RN, MN
VICE PRESIDENT, WILLIAMS & WILKINS

Patricia Feltz Cohen, RN, MA, EdM
CONSULTANT, HUNTINGTON BEACH, CA

Joan Reighley, RN, MN
PSYCHOTHERAPIST, PRIVATE PRACTICE, LOS ANGELES, CA
Certified, specialist; Division of Psychiatric and Mental Health Nursing, American Nurses' Association

A NURSECO BOOK

SANS TACHE

WILLIAMS & WILKINS
Baltimore • London • Los Angeles • Sydney

A NURSECO BOOK
Copyright © 1983—Margo Creighton Neal
Copyright © 1985—Williams & Wilkins
428 East Preston Street, Baltimore, Maryland 21202 U.S.A.

All rights reserved. No part of this book may be reproduced in any form or by any means, including information storage and retrieval systems, without permission in writing from the publisher, except by a reviewer who may quote brief passages in a review.

Printed in the United States of America

Library of Congress Cataloging in Publication Data

Main entry under title:
Nursing care planning guides, set 4, 2nd Ed.

1. Nursing—Handbooks, manuals, etc. 2. Nursing—Planning—Handbooks, manuals, etc. I. Neal, Margo Creighton, 1935–
II. Cohen, Patricia Feltz, 1932– . III. Reighley, Joan, 1936– . IV. Title.
[DNLM: 1. Nursing—Handbooks. 2. Patient care planning—Handbooks. WY 100 N342n 1980]
RT51.N372 1982 610.73 82-14307
ISBN 0-683-09522-6

86 87 88 89 10 9 8 7 6 5 4 3

Set No. 4
TABLE OF CONTENTS

PREFACE

Nursing care plans are the tangible outcomes of the nursing process. These *Nursing Care Planning Guides* are the essence of many nursing care plans. By extrapolating from the Guides what is appropriate for a specific patient, the process of planning patient care and writing care plans becomes a satisfying endeavor. This satisfaction is further reinforced when the nurse evaluates patient response in terms of the written plan and when other staff read and utilize it.

This second edition of *Nursing Care Planning Guides, Set 4,* is part of our continuing effort to provide up-to-date publications for practicing nurses. To achieve this end, we have consulted with many nurses, scanned numerous nursing journals, attended seminars, and synthesized the information into this book. We are gratified by the enormous amount of feedback we have received to our *Nursing Care Planning Guides,* and to know that our efforts are so helpful to nurses writing nursing care plans. More than ever, we are convinced that nurses receive satisfaction from planning and writing nursing care plans—*as long as they have adequate knowledge and tools to guide them*. The *Nursing Care Planning Guides,* based on nursing process, provide that knowledge and tools.

This edition of *Nursing Care Planning Guides, Set 4,* is crossreferenced to the other volumes in this series, Sets 1, 2, 3, and 5. In addition to these five generic sets, we have published clinical editions based on these original sets; e.g., we have pulled all the medical-surgical conditions and published "Nursing Care Planning Guides for Medical-Surgical Care." Other clinical editions available are: Maternity/Pediatrics, Psychiatric/Mental Health, and Long-Term Care.

We have attempted to avoid stereotyping the nurse as "she" and the patient by "he" by using "s/he" in lieu of she/he. However, the English language has yet to produce a combination form for masculine and feminine pronouns; thus you will note some referral to the patient in the masculine form only.

Margo Creighton Neal
Patricia Feltz Cohen
Joan Reighley

INTRODUCTION

To use these Guides to greatest advantage, scan the Table of Contents and select the Guide that is related to a specific patient, for example "The Child with Leukemia." Note its separate components: long-term goal, general considerations, specific considerations, patient outcomes, nursing actions, discharge planning, and recommended references. Review other *Nursing Care Planning Guides* that have been recommended as relating to this content area: "Drugs: Antileukemic," and "The Child who is Dying/Terminal."

Next, assess the patient in terms of the reviewed data, the presenting complaints, sign and symptoms, and behavior. Extrapolate from the Guides essential data that can help you with the next step in the nursing process—making the nursing diagnosis. The "Specific Considerations" section of the Guides contains general areas of nursing diagnosis, such as "Nutrition." To make the diagnosis, choose those specific symptoms/problems that are interfering with the patient's adjustment/recovery, such as *Alteration in nutrition: less than body requirements*; the latter is the nursing diagnosis. Finally, specify expected outcomes for the nursing diagnosis, referring to those suggested in the Guide, using or changing them as appropriate. Next, prescribe nursing actions that will lead to the patient achieving the expected outcomes. Refer to those suggested in the Guides and extrapolate accordingly; add additional ones based on your own nursing judgment. Set a timeframe for evaluating patient response to these interventions: is the patient moving toward the expected outcomes? If not, do you need to review the nursing actions? the outcomes? or is some other nursing diagnosis taking priority? If "yes" to any of these, then revise the plan as needed. Make as many nursing diagnoses, with corresponding outcomes, as necessary. If possible, set a long-term goal; sometimes this cannot be done until the results of diagnostic tests are in.

Consider discharge planning for your patient. What does your patient and/or family/significant other need to know on discharge? Incorporate this teaching into your nursing care plan. To learn more about the content area, read the recommended references that are given.

Use these *Nursing Care Planning Guides* as references and guidelines for planning patient care and writing nursing care plans.

The Patient with an Acute Head Injury

LONG TERM GOAL: The patient will return to home/family/occupational roles with minimal possible residual effects of acute head injury; *OR* the patient will maintain stable vital functions with/without moderate complications and neurological deficits throughout lengthy rehabilitation and convalescence; *OR* the patient will be sustained with compassion and dignity until life support systems have been disconnected; the family will be helped to cope with loss and grief.

General Considerations:

- **Incidence:** over six million head injuries yearly, of which nearly a million are considered to be serious (Glasgow Coma Scale (GCS) Index of less than 8; see Recommended References by Jones, and Connolly and Zewe). In the latter group, there is approximately a 50% mortality rate. Over the age of 20, the chances of a favorable outcome decline with increasing age.
- **Types of acute head injury** include *direct* blow to head (due to impact after a fall or from being hit with an object) or *indirect* by acceleration or deceleration of head due to sudden jolt (often occurs in vehicular collisions). Varieties of head injuries include skull fractures, concussions, cerebral contusions, lacerations, edema, and cerebral hemorrhage (subarachnoid bleeding; brainstem bleeding; subdural, epidural, or intracerebral hematomas).
- **Concussion** is the term used for the minor, temporary loss of brain function caused by tissue shock from a jarring of the brain; severe brain damage is not present and there is a spontaneous recovery of all neurological functions within a couple of days. *Common presenting signs* of a concussion include amnesia, confusion, change in vision and equilibrium, and loss of consciousness lasting less than 24 hours. There may be a postconcussion syndrome, lasting for several weeks, characterized by headaches, dizziness, anxiety, fatigue, inability to concentrate, and emotional lability. Impaired memory and delayed reaction times are also commonly reported.
- **Contusions** involve structural alterations of the brain, longer periods of unconsciousness (compared to concussion), and residual neurological impairment. Cerebral lacerations and bleeding also cause serious sequelae. Cerebral edema is a swelling of the brain tissue within a closed cranium resulting in increased intracranial pressure (IIP), which, if not promptly reduced, leads to brain damage and death.
- **Consequences of head injury** range from no neurological disturbance to a persistent vegetative state, or death; therefore every head injury must be considered potentially serious and possibly complicated by other injuries to vital organs or iatrogenic trauma from improper treatment. Head injuries are also more serious when associated with alcohol and/or drug abuse because accurate neurological assessment is more difficult when signs are masked or potentiated.

- **Diagnostic measures** include complete neurological history and physical exam; computerized tomography (CT) scans (see Recommended References) and x-rays (skull films and cervical spine series to level of C-7 and T-1, at least; chest x-ray, IVP, and other x-rays for possible internal injuries); echoencephalography and cerebral angiography (see NCPG #5:04, "The Patient Needing Angiography") are sometimes used for evaluating possible hematoma.
- **Treatment** aims to assess accurately and to diagnose quickly the nature of the head injury and its consequences; to prevent or promptly control cerebral bleeding, edema, increased intracranial pressure, and brain damage; and to provide correct, expert medical and nursing measures for the maintenance of vital functions and for the promotion of brain healing. Treatment may include intracranial surgery (see NCPG #4:12, "The Patient Undergoing Intracranial Surgery"). Long-term convalescent care and complete rehabilitation is planned by specialists for those patients with critical head injuries who survive. Residual effects of spasticity, seizures, persistent neurological deficits, and psycho/social/emotional disturbances may be encountered. The outlook for improvement over time is better for children than for adults.
- Major **immediate nursing responsibilities** include (1) ensuring an open airway and adequate respiratory function to prevent hypoxia and hypercarbia (which raise IIP); (2) maintaining circulating blood volume and adequate cardiac output; (3) ascertaining neurological status as soon as possible and keeping neurological assessment records (a comprehensive, useful neurological observation record form and performance check list to assure inter-rater reliability are both highly desirable; see Recommended References to develop an improved one for your hospital); (4) obtaining as accurate and complete as possible history of the injury, its effects, any treatment received, and any previous relevant history (diseases, medications, allergies, etc.) from patient, family member, friend, or witness to accident; (5) planning, implementing, and evaluating medical therapy and nursing care to prevent and control IIP; (6) preparing patient (and family) for surgery, if indicated; and (7) providing explanations and realistic reassurance to patient and family.

Specific Considerations, Potential Patient Outcomes, and Nursing Actions:

1) Neurological Observation and Assessment

The patient's neurological status will be continually monitored for changes indicating a need for intervention; early signs of IIP will be identified and reported immediately:

- arrange for 1-to-1 (if possible) primary care in a neurological ICU to provide reliable, consistent, competent neurological observations & assessments;
- see this section in NCPG #4:11, "The Patient with Actual/Potential Increased Intracranial Pressure;"
- know the different levels of consciousness (LOC) & describe pt.'s behavior clearly, carefully, & comprehensively, unless your hospital uses an exceptionally reliable, standardized, neurological observation record; ob-

tain frequent (Q15 minutes) & continuing checks of LOC;

— check for symmetry & strength of reflexes & note presence or absence (gag, swallow, elbow, knees, Babinski);

— check ability to speak without hoarseness or dysphasia;

— observe, record, & report (during succeeding days of hospitalization) aftereffects of head injury such as headache, nausea, vomiting, dizziness, emotional irritability; record type of amnesia (retrograde—events prior to injury; antegrade—events during & following injury); note presence & type of aphasia or dysphasia;

— note & report bruising behind ear (Battle's sign), periorbital ecchymosis ("racoon eyes"), otorrhea, or rhinorrhea (either bleeding or CSF);

— do not elevate pt.'s head or flex neck until spinal injury has been ruled out (cervical collar may be temporarily applied until cervical spine films are taken & diagnosis is clear); examine pt. for scalp wounds, skull lumps, or tenderness; look for CSF leakage from nose & ears; smell for alcohol on pt.'s breath (this may confuse neurological assessment but not all symptoms may be alcohol-related); review & assess function of cranial nerves;

— accompany pt. for CT scan in order to provide constant, consistent nursing care & monitoring, especially if pt. is a child or an adult in critical condition; explain to pt. (if possible) & family what this painless, though frightening, procedure entails; give necessary prescribed presedation & remain with pt. to note & record response;

— ask pt./family member/friend/witness to the injury about the:

a) cause of injury (a missile? object striking the head? fall? auto or vehicular collision? sudden jolt?);

b) site of injury, direction and force of blow, secondary injury resulting from fall after blow;

c) any loss of consciousness? for what length of time? how aroused? any seizures before or after fall or head injury? if so, obtain as complete a description as possible; length of time since injury; behavior since injury (level of alertness or responsiveness);

d) other signs & symptoms such as bleeding from ears, nose, eyes, mouth, or elsewhere; clear fluid leakage from nose, ears, head; paralysis, loss of feeling, limpness or weakness of extremities; loss of bladder or bowel control; signs of infection; signs of fluid imbalance; vomiting; headache; amnesia, aphasia, or dysphasia;

e) treatment, drugs, alcohol taken before injury or exact treatment or medications administered before arrival at hospital after injury; history of frequent accidents, falls, head injuries, seizures, or illnesses.

2) Maintenance of Vital Functions and Prevention of Complications

The patient will maintain adequate respiratory function, fluid & electrolyte balance, cardiac output, and elimination; the patient will be free of infection and preventable complications resulting from immobility and therapeutic regimen; the patient will be monitored continuously for early signs of IIP:

— see this section in NCPG #4:11, "The Patient with Actual/Potential Increased Intracranial Pressure;"
— elevate head of bed 15°–30° to promote cerebral venous drainage by gravity;
— aspirate blood, mucus, or vomitus PRN; remove loose teeth; start O_2 to prevent cerebral hypoxia & further brain damage; control ventilation PRN to regulate accumulation of CO_2 in blood (hypercarbia or hypercapnia), which will cause cerebral vessel dilation resulting in congestion & increased ICP; have tracheostomy set & mechanical ventilator ready; endotracheal intubation will probably be indicated for accompanying severe chest trauma, inadequate respiration, or deteriorating neurological status (GCS Index of 8 or less);
— know that the side-lying position is usually preferred for the comatose pt. to prevent aspiration & airway occlusion, but location & extent of injuries may alter this; maintain functional body alignment; avoid neck flexion (increases IIP); avoid hip flexion (increases intra-abdominal pressure leading to increased IIP); turn pt. slowly & gently, log-rolling to keep body straight; have pt. exhale while turning to prevent Valsalva maneuver (breath holding that increases intrathoracic & intra-abdominal pressure);
— insert an NG tube as appropriate; if NG tube in place, keep patent; check for GI bleeding & know that ulceration is possible from stress or from glucocorticosteroids; give antacids Q2H & cimetidine as prescribed;
— know that, except for cases of hypovolemic shock, fluid intake will be restricted (sometimes to 600–1000 ml/24 hours); use microdrip IV tubing sets & monitor rate of parenteral therapy closely;
— check vital signs Q15 minutes; check for signs of bleeding & blood loss; assess for internal & external injuries & signs of hypovolemic shock; establish IV lines for parenteral administration of glucose, blood, Ringers Lactate, volume expanders, etc.; place pt. on cardiac monitor; maintain arterial lines for blood gas determinations & monitoring; obtain specimens for necessary lab work (CBC, Hct., Hbg., T&C, etc.);
— assist lab & x-ray personnel with necessary tests so pt. is not moved or disturbed unnecessarily or harmfully;
— protect pt. from injuries due to restless movements, disorientation, & seizures, but avoid physical restraints unless absolutely necessary & ordered (fighting & restlessness increase ICP); assess, report, & attempt to correct causes of restlessness (pain, a distended bladder due to a kinked or clamped catheter, tight casts or

bandages, respiratory distress, bleeding, increasing ICP); if pt. is regaining consciousness s/he may need a member of the family or close friend to be there; there is evidence to indicate that if they hold pt.'s hand, stroke pt., or talk to pt., this causes a drop in ICP & pt. will be calmer; avoid unnecessary sedation that may cause respiratory depression & mask neurological symptoms;

— prevent contractures with standard measures (bed board, foot board, trochanter rolls, & devices to prevent hand deformities); give passive range-of-motion exercises (isometric exercises will increase ICP); understand & cooperate with physical therapy aims & program;

— bathe & inspect skin QD for hydration & turgor, rashes, abrasions, contusions; signs of pressure sores, infection or phlebitis at puncture sites; give soothing sensory stimulation by stroking & touching while talking to pt.;

— use standard decubitus-prevention measures (alternating pressure pad or flotation mattress); give massage & protection for heels, elbows, & bony prominences, etc.;

— give mouth care Q2-4H with saline or peroxide swabs (glycerin may increase crusting); clean tongue & teeth; apply cream to nostrils & lips;

— pad side rails & take seizure precautions especially if pt. has a seizure history, a skull fracture, a suspected hematoma, or a GCS score of 8 or less; have parenteral forms of diphenylhydantoin (Dilantin) & diazepam (Valium) (drug of choice for status epilepticus) readily available; know that the therapeutic blood level loading dose of 10 mg/Kg will last about 24 hours;

— if steroids are used to reduce cerebral edema, watch for associated side effects; see NCPG #5:43, "Drugs: Corticosteroids;" know that fluid & electrolyte balance will be more difficult to manage & pt. must be watched closely for signs of infection other than inflammation;

— keep close family members & friends honestly informed of pt.'s progress, prognosis, & current plan of treat ment; encourage them to assist with pt. care whenever possible & to spend as much time as possible with pt., to talk with pt., to play pt.'s favorite music or inspirational tape recordings for stimulation; remind them that pt. can often hear & understand, that pts. are soothed by familiar voices & sounds;

— encourage pt.'s family & friends to express their fears, feelings of helplessness, guilt, anger, & despair outside the pt.'s hearing range; arrange for spiritual & emotional counseling PRN;

— support *realistic* hopes (1 study showed only 6% of patients with coma lasting longer than 2 months made any significant recovery, but there are surprising exceptions); prepare them for the prolonged care usually associated with serious head-injured pts., i.e., long-term recovery & rehabilitation; help them to think through the decisions regarding practical arrangements & adjustments that must be made for each member of the pt.'s nuclear family.

3) Patient/Family Education — The family/significant other will know observations of patient to make at home; will know signs of untoward developments:

— instruct to awaken pt. Q1–2H x 24 hours and ask pt. to state own name, where s/he is, & what happened;
— tell them to bring pt. to emergency dept. *immediately* for
- *severe* headache (give only aspirin or acetaminophen for headaches, nothing stronger; do not give alcohol, tranquilizers, antihistamines, or other medications);
- *persistent* vomiting (mild nausea & vomiting are common; give clear liquids & soups as tolerated for 1st 24 hours after head injury);
- unequal pupils or vacant, staring look in pt.'s eyes;
- weakness, limpness, or loss of feeling in arms or legs; any kind of seizure or stiffness in body;
- any drainage from nose or ears.

Discharge Planning and Teaching Objectives/Outcomes:

1) (Patient/Family/Significant Other) Can state the normal aftereffects of an acute, *minor* head injury (headache; dizziness; *some* drowsiness and fatigue; emotional irritability and periodic euphoria or depression; difficulty speaking, remembering, computing sums, writing paragraphs) and knows that these may last from a few days to a month or longer. Knows that impaired memory and delayed reaction time also may follow even a minor head injury and patient should return to former activities gradually and part-time.
2) Knows that following a *moderate* head injury, in addition to above symptoms, patient may also have episodes of hallucinations, delusions, personality alterations, cognitive disorders, sleep disturbances, and psychosocial disturbances for many months to years (over the years, most of these sequelae eventually disappear).
3) Knows (has been told) if there is a risk of seizures, so that activities of daily living can be adjusted accordingly, if desired.
4) (If patient is to be sent home instead of to a convalescent hospital or rehabilitation center) Has reviewed a written plan for permitted activities, exercise, diet, medication, and rehabilitation. Family is well prepared to provide appropriate care for physical

and emotional needs of convalescing patient.

5) Can identify signs of *increasing* difficulty (irrational behavior changed from pre-injury behavior, restlessness, combativeness, amnesia, disorientation, *increasing* limb weakness and difficulty walking or speaking, *increasing* drowsiness and unresponsiveness to verbal commands). Knows to seek immediate medical care without further delay.
6) Has medical appointment for follow-up medical and psychologic rehabilitation and care.
7) If needed, has received social service referral for assistance with arrangements for disability income, homemaker service, child care arrangements, community health nursing services, physical, speech, or occupational therapy, and psychologic counseling.

Recommended References

"Acute Head Injury: What To Do When . . . And Why," by J. Kunkel and J. Wiley. *Nursing 79*, March 1979:23–33.

"Bringing the Unconscious Patient Back Safely—Nursing Makes the Critical Difference," by N. Mauss-Clum. *Nursing 82*, August 1982:34–42.

"Computed Tomographic Scanning of the Brain," NIH Consensus Development Conference Summary. Bethesda, MD: National Institute of Neurological and Communicative Disorders and Stroke (20205), November, 1981.

"Concussion," by C. Fritz. *Nursing 81*, September 1981:84.

"Drugs: Corticosteroids." *NCP Guide #5:43*, Nurseco, 1981.

"Glasgow Coma Scale," by C. Jones. *American Journal of Nursing*, September 1979:1551–1553.

"Head Injuries. Part 1, Advances in Care During Past Decade," "Part 2, Advances in Diagnostic Equipment," by J. Young. *Nursing Times*, April 30, 1981:766–769; May 7, 1981:819–821.

"Head Trauma." *Emergency Medicine*, November 15, 1980:103–105.

"Life-Threatening Head and Spinal Injuries," by P. Perdue. *RN*, June 1981:36–41.

"Nursing Management of the Head Injured Patient," by J. Kunkel. *Critical Care Update*, March 1981:22–24.

"Of Course You Can Manage Head Trauma Patients," by K. Mastrian. *RN*, August 1981:44–51.

"Outcome Following Closed Head Injury," by C. Jones. *The Journal of Neurosurgical Nursing*, August 1981:178–183.

"The Patient with Actual/Potential Increased Intracranial Pressure." *NCP Guide #4:11*, 2nd Ed., Nurseco, 1983.

"The Patient Needing Angiography." *NCP Guide #5:04*, Nurseco, 1981.

"The Patient Undergoing Intracranial Surgery." *NCP Guide #4:12*, 2nd Ed., Nurseco, 1983.

"Traumatic Head Injury: Restlessness and Agitation as Prognosticators of Physical and Psychological Improvement in Patients," by R. Reyes et al. *Archives of Physical Medicine and Rehabilitation*, January 1981:20–23.

"Update: Head Injuries," by R. Connolly and G. Zewe. *Journal of Neurosurgical Nursing*, August 1981:195–201.

"What To Say . . . And Do . . . When Your Patient Asks About CT Scans," by C. Haughey. *Nursing 81*, December 1981:72–77.

The Patient with an Amputation

Definition: Amputation is the traumatic or surgical removal of an appendage or limb.

LONG TERM GOAL: The patient will recover from the amputation of a limb free of preventable complications; the patient will accept an altered body image and adapt effectively to use of a prosthesis; within necessary limitations, the patient will return to near normal roles in home/job/community after a reasonable rehabilitation period.

General Considerations:

— **Indications:** amputation of any limb or digit may be needed to resolve congenital deformities, tumors, traumatic injuries, chronic infections, or problems related to peripheral vascular disease. *NOTE:* the principles of this nursing guide apply to the loss of any limb, but will be especially applicable to the more common occurrence, the loss of a lower limb.

— **Nursing responsibilities** include pre- and postoperative care; refer to NCPGs #2:44, "General Pre-op Care," and #s 2:41–43, "General Post-op Care, Parts A, B, and C." Early ambulation via crutches, walker, or temporary prosthesis is usually emphasized. The nurse plays a major role in assisting the patient and family to accept the loss and to participate actively in a vigorous rehabilitation program aimed at complete self-respect and self-reliance. Together they set realistic activities of daily living (ADL) goals and coordinate the program suggested by physician, physical therapist, occupational therapist, and recreational therapist (rehabilitation team). They may wish to use the rehabilitation classification below for goal setting.

— **Rusk Classification of Rehabilitation** (see Recommended References):

1) *Full restoration*: handicapped client, but not disabled
2) *Partial restoration*: needs some modification of former activities
3) *Self-care plus*: can work and take care of self with only some modifications
4) *Self-care minus*: needs help with ADL and with ambulation
5) *Cosmetic plus*: cannot ambulate; has prosthesis for psychologic reasons
6) *Not feasible*: no prosthesis; confined to a wheelchair.

— Whether inevitable and planned or traumatic and unforeseen, in our society amputation is a catastrophic blow to the individual. The level and satisfaction of successful rehabilitation depends not only on the skill of the rehabilitation team, but to a large extent on the premorbid personality, physical and psychologic strengths of the amputee, along with adequacy of the family and friend support systems that are available. Since most lower-limb amputations are performed because of occlusive peripheral vascular disease, the patient is usually older, often a smoker, and has a complicating medical condition such as diabetes or cardiovascular disease. A second amputation, higher on the affected limb or on the previously unoperated limb, may be necessary. These complicating factors necessitate a vigorous rehabilitation plan that is nevertheless *realistic* in terms of the individual patient.

Specific Considerations, Potential Patient Outcomes, and Nursing Actions:

1) Pre-op Preparation

The patient will provide informed consent for amputation; the patient will express fears, anxieties, feelings, and questions associated with the impending amputation; the patient will participate in muscle-strengthening exercises preparatory to use of prosthesis; the patient will be physically prepared for a successful surgical outcome; the patient will know what to expect postoperatively regarding type of stump dressing or cast and prospects for early ambulation with a temporary prosthesis:

— know what the MD has told the pt./family; correct distorted & confused information caused by anxiety & selective inattention; provide as much information as they want;
— be aware that the grieving process is triggered as soon as the decision to amputate is made; tell pt. that other amputees have had feelings & questions that needed to be expressed, so pt. may wish to share these with you; allocate time for this purpose;
— explain about the post-op stump dressing or cast after learning surgeon's plans for this pt.;
— if pre-op time permits, have pt. do sit-ups, pull-ups (with trapeze), and active-resistance exercises to develop muscle strength for post-op rehabilitation;
— administer prophylactic antibiotics as ordered;
— see NCPG #2:44, "General Pre-op Care," for additional nursing considerations.

2) Post-op Measures

The patient will resume normal cardiopulmonary function with fluids and electrolytes in balance; the patient will be free of preventable complications; the patient will maintain an adequate output with normal elimination restored:

— position pt. as ordered, usually with the foot of the bed elevated, in a post-op orthopedic bed, complete with bed board, foot board (or cradle), & trapeze;
— monitor & record TPR & BP, according to standard post-op routine, until stable, then Q8H, noting & reporting temperature elevations of 2 or more degrees after the 3rd post-op day;
— monitor & record I&O carefully, accurately;
— monitor IV fluids PRN; progress to a regular or special diet as tolerated when ordered; emphasize foods con-

taining Vitamin C & protein to promote wound healing; administer vitamin & mineral supplements as ordered;
- administer analgesics PRN;
- protect bony prominences of sacrum & unoperated limbs from pressure sores; know these areas suffer "shear" abrasion from "scooting" up & down in bed;
- check voiding Q4H; notify MD if voiding frequent, small amounts or if unable to void 6 hours post-op when intake has been adequate;
- check elimination, giving laxatives PRN when solid food intake is reestablished;
- assist pt. to sit up on side of bed, dangle, then get up on the 1st post-op day, as soon as permitted;
- turn, cough, & deep breathe Q2H while on bedrest;
- for additional nursing actions, see NCPGs #2:41–43, "General Post-op Nursing Care, Parts A, B, & C."

3) Stump Care — The patient's stump will heal without infection or flexion contracture; edema will subside and the residual limb size will be reduced:
- during 1st 24 hours post-op, elevate stump by elevating foot of bed;
- apply ice bags; observe & report excessive bleeding or edema; reinforce dressing PRN; measure & record Hemovac drainage, taking care to maintain position & patency of tubes;
- after 1st 2 hours, position pt. on side, back, or abdomen with stump in correctly EXTENDED alignment (no pillows or flexion permitted); keep pt. on abdomen at least 2–3 hours/shift to stretch flexor muscles & prevent contractures;
- when pt. is ready & if cast not in place, proceed slowly to teach pt. to dress & wrap own stump, usually Q4H, to help shape stump & to reduce edema; position a mirror for easier visibility; use aseptic technique; cleanse & dry skin thoroughly; demonstrate "figure eight" wrapping pattern (never circular direction) with elastic bandages, applying even tension across the distal end of the stump to shape stump for proper prosthesis fit; know that shrinker socks may be used for more effective reduction of residual limb volume, teach pt. how to apply these properly;
- once each shift, at least, provide full range-of-motion exercises to all normal limbs & joints; see NCPG #1:47, "Range of Motion Exercises;" pay special attention to affected limb; if a below-knee amputation, supervise quadriceps muscle-setting exercise QID; teach pt. to perform abdominal & buttocks muscle-setting exercise to improve strength for balanced walking; do not rely totally on physical therapy sessions to strengthen & limber pt. muscles; observe physical therapy & reinforce teaching with regular, short practice sessions;

— to increase circulation to stump, get pt. out of bed as often as possible, beginning on the 1st or 2nd post-op day; elevate & protect stump while up in chair; do not allow stump to remain in a fixed or dependent position for more than 1 hour; assist pt. to walk with crutches, walker, temporary prosthesis, etc.; have a regular shoe on unaffected leg to provide good balance & support; teach tightening of buttock & abdominal muscles to help in standing & balancing.

4) Psychosocial Adjustment (to Loss of Limb, Altered Body Image, Use of Prosthesis, Temporary Dependency, Pain)

The patient will demonstrate adaptive acceptance of loss, mobilizing emotional and psychic energy to gain independence and actively participate in rehabilitation program; the patient will experience and express relief of fears, anxiety, depression, discouragement, and pain; the patient will achieve and express a sense of self-reliance and self-respect; the patient will retain responsibility for actions, decisions, and as many aspects of self-care as feasible:

— provide time & opportunities for pt. & family to talk, ask questions, express feelings, & relive the immediate past experiences that they wish to discuss; focus on what they share with you & do not challenge the validity according to your perceptions; know that they will need to ventilate feelings on more than 1 occasion throughout rehabilitation; refer to NCPGs #1:31, "Responses to Loss," & #2:29, "The Patient Experiencing a Body Image Disturbance;"
— recognize & help pt. & family to see that disability usually causes feelings of depression, anger, hostility, resentment, frustration, helplessness, & hopelessness; help them to constructively channel the energy associated with such feelings by increasing self-care & decision-making activities;
— know that a period of denial is expected during adaptation to a loss (may take the form of refusing to look at stump or change dressing); accept the denial but do not support it;
— talk with other nursing staff about maintaining a consistent attitude & approach with pt. & family; try to be patient, understanding, positive, & firm;
— discuss pt.'s adjustment with family & friends, urge them to support, encourage, applaud all positive efforts to cope/adapt; praise their efforts to help, but remind them that pt. must be allowed as much control of his life as possible; even if pt. must be physically or financially dependent, s/he should be helped to see that responsibility as an adult includes not only helping self, but showing consideration for others;
— accept the pt.'s description of true surgical *or* phantom limb pain/sensation/discomfort/spasm; pt. may also experience fear, anxiety, restlessness; provide analgesics, sedatives, and/or tranquilizers PRN as ordered; know that sometimes pressure, heat, whirlpool, or visualizing muscle relaxation can help reduce phantom limb pain & spasm; explain that phantom limb sensations ("dull," "sharp," "shooting," "cramping," "burn-

ing," "tingling," etc.) are normal & to be expected, that they may last over a period of many months; know that pts. need to be prepared for these unpleasant sensations, but try to explain it in a matter-of-fact manner as the psyche "catching up" with the body change; teach pt. that stress-management techniques & increased activity (physical, mental, & social) will help him to cope when drugs are no longer feasible;

— if possible, have a successfully adjusted amputee visit the pt. & family to share experiences, to inspire courage & hope, and to provide practical information about use of a prosthesis.

5) Adaptation to Prosthesis The patient will wear prosthesis with confidence and skill; the patient will state s/he knows that discomfort, fatigue, and awkwardness are to be expected and are temporary; the patient will express optimism and determination to achieve satisfactory fit and prosthetic usage:

— remind pt. & family that the early, temporary prosthesis will not be attractive or "normal" in appearance, but that the final version will more nearly resemble the "real thing;" tell them it will also be better fitting, more comfortable, & easier to use;

— observe prosthetist's teaching session; know how prosthesis should be worn, handled, maintained so you can reinforce teaching realistically & practically;

— see that pt. applies sock & liner smoothly without wrinkles; have clean, spare ones available; remind pt. to use only clean, dry ones daily;

— teach pt. to watch stump for signs of skin irritation, redness, warmth, tenderness; clean skin with mild soap & water daily, dry skin thoroughly; avoid lubricating ointment or creams that soften skin, unless skin is very dry & scaly;

— urge pt. to wear prosthesis through early periods of discomfort & awkwardness; help him keep records of increasing tolerance; have pt. set realistic goals for self, but don't permit quitting after temporary setbacks;

— remind family that throughout rehabilitation, there may be periods of sleep disturbance, anorexia, weight loss, withdrawal, & other signs of anxiety/depression; urge them to maintain a positive, encouraging attitude of support;

— know & tell pt./family that amputees with vascular disease may not be fitted with a prosthesis for several months post-op until healing is assured & shrinkage is satisfactorily achieved; teach appropriate aseptic dressing changes & stump care to be done at home (or write out procedure for nursing home personnel);

— check your local community for mutual aid support group providing telephone counseling and personal help or contact The Mutual Aid Foundation for Amputees, 5833 Costello Ave., Van Nuys, CA, 213/988-1666.

Discharge Planning and Teaching Objectives/Outcomes

1) (Patient/Family/Significant Other) Demonstrates correct application and care of prosthesis. Has written instructions. Plans to keep regular appointments (every four to six weeks) with prosthetist as long as needed.
2) Has an appointment for follow-up medical care with family physician as well as for orthopedic or rehabilitation clinic.
3) With prosthesis, demonstrates ability to stand, balance, walk, climb, get up from a fall, and maintain good posture and balance in a variety of situations. If no prosthesis or if a bilateral amputee, has learned to use a wheelchair safely and effectively with appropriate transfer techniques.
4) Demonstrates muscle strengthening exercises not only for residual limb muscles but for rest of body as well. States s/he recognizes need to continue conditioning exercises for optimal well-being and rehabilitation.
5) Demonstrates proper stump care; knows to consult physician and prosthetist promptly for stump redness, tenderness, infection, or problems of prosthetic fit, comfort, and control. Knows the stump will continue to shrink for up to two years.
6) Has a referral name & number for assistance with social security, disability insurance, homemaker service, home health nursing, physical therapy, and, if possible, another long-time, successfully rehabilitated amputee (or amputee group) willing to help.

Recommended References

"Amputation," by J. Iveson-Iveson. *Nursing Mirror*, June 24, 1981:34, 35.
"Amputation: Two Views," by B. Buck and A. Lee. *Nursing Clinics of North America*, December 1976:641–657.
"Battered Body—A Teenage Amputee Taught Us Four Tips For Better Long-Term Care," by L. Wiley et al. *Nursing 78*, January 1978:36–41.
"Care of the Amputee Patient," by P. Delfeld. *Journal of Nursing Care*, October 1981:16–17.
"Comparing the Effectiveness of Elastic Bandages and Shrinker Socks for Lower Extremity Amputees," by K. Manella. *Physical Therapy*, March 1981:334–337.
"Coping With a Leg Amputation," by J. Walters. *American Journal of Nursing*, July 1981:1349–1352.
"General Postoperative Nursing Care, Parts A, B, and C." *NCP Guides #2:41–43,* 2nd Ed., Nurseco, 1980.
"General Preoperative Nursing Care." *NCP Guide #2:44*, 2nd Ed., Nurseco, 1980.
"Learning To Live With A New Leg," by R. Meador. *American Journal of Nursing*, August 1979:1393–1395.
"Nursing of the Upper Extremity Amputee and Preparation for Prosthetic Training," by V. McClinton. *Nursing Clinics of North America*, December 1976:659–669.
"Range of Motion Exercises." *NCP Guide #1:47*, 2nd Ed., Nurseco, 1980.
"Rehabilitation of the Patient with a Lower Extremity Amputation," by J. Engstrand. *Nursing Clinics of North America*, December 1976:659–669.
Rehabilitation Medicine, 4th Ed., by H. Rusk. St. Louis: Mosby 1977:407, 408.
"Responses to Loss: The Grief and Mourning Process." *NCP Guide #1:31*, 2nd Ed., Nurseco, 1980.
"The Last Resort," by P. Datta. *Nursing Mirror*, March 10, 1982:41–43.
"The Patient Experiencing a Body Image Disturbance." *NCP Guide #2:29*, 2nd Ed., Nurseco, 1980.
"The Patient Experiencing Pain." *NCP Guide #1:30*, 2nd Ed., Nurseco, 1980.
"Unique Treatment Approach for a Patient with a Below-the-Knee Amputation," by M. Amstutz. *Physical Therapy*, January 1981:37–39.

The Patient with Aphasia/Dysphasia

Definition: *Aphasia* is the conventional general term used for labeling organic-caused losses or disturbances in language (reading, writing, understanding, and speaking-usage of symbolic signs and sounds) due to cerebral damage. *Dysphasia* is partial speech impairment (this term is more correct, but "aphasia" is more commonly used).

LONG TERM GOAL: The patient will recover optimum language skills over time (six months to two years). S/he will experience self-respect and seek opportunities to initiate social interactions.

General Considerations:

— **Incidence and occurrence:** an estimated 1 million persons in the US suffer from aphasia.

— **Types of aphasia** include

- *Global*: a total inability to formulate, understand, or express language symbols; reflects severe, extensive, generalized brain dysfunction.
- *Receptive* (also called sensory, fluent, or Wernicke's): a loss in ability to understand the spoken word (auditory-comprehension deficit) or the written word (reading-comprehension deficit). Patients with auditory-comprehension deficit cannot monitor the words they say or recognize their errors of speech. They often substitute words or sounds in error, making their speech meaningless. In milder cases, patients may be aware of their incorrect speech and become frustrated, concerned, and depressed.
- *Expressive* (also called motor, nonfluent, or Broca's): a loss in ability to speak effectively, using appropriate words and sentences. The causative lesion is in the motor-association area known as Broca's area. These patients have little or no auditory- or reading-comprehension problems and are therefore very much aware of their spoken language problems; they are frequently very depressed and frustrated.
- *Anomic* (or amnesic): the inability to recall correct names for objects, people, places, or events. The usual cause is a lesion in the area of the brain thought to hold learned associations.
- *Mixed, nonfluent*: a disorder involving both expressive and auditory comprehension deficits.
- *Conduction*: characterized by literal paraphasia, but comprehension is intact; the lesion is present in the bundle of fibers connecting Broca's area to Wernicke's area.

— **Diagnostic terms** commonly used include
- *Dyslexia:* difficulty understanding reading material.
- *Dysgraphia:* difficulty writing words or sentences and composing coherent paragraphs.
- *Dysarthria*: impaired articulation; the speech-producing muscles and nerves are damaged.
- *Verbal dyspraxia*: inability to form the mouth and tongue movements properly to pronounce a word, even though the muscles are normal and the idea of the word is clearly understood.
- *Literal paraphasia*: substitution of incorrect sounds.
- *Verbal paraphasia*: substitution of one word for another.

— **Cause** of aphasia (all types) is most often a CVA, but occurs in other forms of cerebral trauma, with space-occupying lesions, infections, or toxic-agent poisoning (such as lead). Aphasia normally results from damage to left cerebral hemisphere (believed to be the area of language for most people); the degree of severity and the pattern of deficit vary according to the location of the affected part of the brain.

— **Prognosis:** the potential for recovery depends on a number of influencing variables, including the cause and extent of damage; the length of time ensuing before adequate retraining occurs; the age, general physical and mental health, educational level, intelligence, character, and motivation of the patient; the extent of involvement and help from family and friends. The best chance of improving the language impairment is during the first six months following injury; time should not be lost once the acute phase is over and the patient is medically stable.

— **Assessment** of aphasia is sometimes made using the *Schuell Classification*, ranging from Group 1 (those with simple minor language impairment) through Group 5 (complete, probably irreversible loss of language skills).

— **Evaluation of language losses** and speech retraining is best performed by a qualified speech pathologist. For a list of those professionals, write: American Speech-Language-Hearing Association, 10801 Rockville Pike, Rockville, MD 20852.

— **Nursing responsibilities** include observing and describing the pattern and extent of language deficits in conjunction with family members and friends. A basic assessment of speech status is desirable, describing the extent of the patient's abilities to comprehend spoken and written language, to name objects, to repeat spoken language, to express oneself verbally, and to write meaningful sentences. Much can be accomplished by obtaining learning aids and referring to recommended references. Nurse, patient, and family need to set a goal, make a plan, and practice, practice, practice! When available, professional training in a speech clinic or rehabilitation center is desirable.

Specific Considerations, Potential Patient Outcomes, and Nursing Actions:

1) Talking to Aphasic Patients

The patient will receive verbal input (auditory stimulation) from nurse, therapist, family, and friends that is aimed at restoring lost language skills; the patient will be assisted to communicate his basic needs; the patient will participate in short, well-planned therapeutic language sessions within the limits of his physical and psychologic endurance:

— attract the attention of the pt. by using his name; then face him directly with sufficient light on you for pt. to see your facial movements & body language; be sure to stand on the *unimpaired* side of a stroke pt. to accommodate visual-field cut;

— most aphasics prefer speech at an ordinary conversation level without extraneous sounds in the room (TV, radio, corridor noises, machines, more than 1 speaking at a time, etc.); adjust voice level to the individual; a common error is to shout or raise one's voice as if that would facilitate understanding;

— speak *slower* & more distinctly than normal, retaining facial expressions, feeling tones, gestures, & nonverbal cues to meaning; know that, for severely aphasic persons, studies show combined method of verbal & pantomime instruction works better than 1 method alone; demonstrate, with humor & patience, while speaking clearly & slowly, such examples as "open your mouth," "make a fist," "wash your face," "turn your head," "drink from the glass," "cough," etc.;

— use short phrases; ask only 1 simple question at a time; avoid long sentences & overtalking; it is OK, even advisable, to repeat, *but* make certain the need is clearly indicated; pause to allow time for pt. to process, comprehend, formulate, & give a response;

— to improve effectiveness, plan to do communications evaluation & speech training or teaching in the morning before physical therapy & other fatiguing activities; be sure that pt. is somewhat relaxed & not upset over something else before beginning a learning session; provide privacy to avoid embarrassment;

— be careful to validate level of understanding when relaying specific, important information; know that all aphasics have *some* difficulty understanding the spoken word, but because of reliance on visual & situational cues, they are *likely to understand more* than their speech output might indicate; don't make false or premature assumptions even with those pts. having severe receptive aphasia; if there is a misunderstanding, let pt. know it, don't ignore it, correct it patiently, & go on to something else;

— help the pt. feel less isolated & withdrawn by maintaining him in a social environment; urge visitors & other pts. to persist in their efforts to communicate; encourage them to read the newspaper or mail to pt.; have them describe the weather, sporting events, current news stories, or ward happenings;
— consult with speech therapist to promote cooperation & a consistent approach; encourage all who come in contact with pt. to remain cheerful & optimistic; emphasize capabilities & reinforce pt.'s sense of self-esteem; expect the pt. to feel frustrated & depressed from time to time; acknowledge this feeling & indicate your understanding & acceptance;
— remember that aphasia does *not* mean intellectual impairment or personality degeneration; aphasics are people with brains, feelings, opinions, & rights; they need explanations & information; don't talk about them to the staff or to visitors as if they weren't present or unable to understand you; treat them as adults with respect & dignity; recognize that they have a right to make decisions about their care & should be allowed to participate in life around them as they wish.

2) Listening to Aphasic Patients

The patient will verbally express requests, feelings, etc., to an understanding, patient listener (nurse/therapist/family member):
— *take time* to listen until the pt. is finished speaking; avoid nervous mannerisms (drumming fingers, tapping feet, etc.) or any signs of impatience (sighs, tight mouth, etc.); allow for the extra time that this type of pt. will need; don't interrupt;
— many aphasics appreciate your finishing a sentence for them at times, especially in the early weeks of training, but at least 1 in 3 does not; ask the pt. which s/he prefers & be guided by the response; if s/he has word-finding difficulty (common among all types of aphasics), try supplying 2 or 3 word choices, but only after pt. has been unsuccessful a couple of times; if you are sure of the word, try giving the pt. an open-ended sentence to use to practice the word;
— do not pretend to understand when you don't; aphasics sense this & shut up; some people suggest that you not indicate when you don't comprehend, so that the pt. does not feel rejected or depressed—but honesty with understanding & compassion is a more desirable approach;
— try guessing several possibilities; say, "do you mean . . . ?";
— ask pt. to "talk around the subject" (called circumlocution) to give you clues about the word; say, "how do you use it?"; sometimes you can make it a game (e.g., "Is it bigger than a watermelon or smaller than an orange?");

- don't ask a pt. to write a word s/he cannot say; often the impairment is similar (could you write the name of something you couldn't think of?);
- create & use a book showing pictures of familiar items; help pt. name these;
- speech may be slurred, but if the word is right, then accept the faulty pronunciation; finding the right word is 1 step of progress; when the pt. speaks more freely, you can begin correcting mistakes;
- as pt. regains speech, ask him to talk about topics that are familiar, important, & interesting to him (e.g., present or former job, family, hobby, sports, cooking, gardening, music, etc.);
- let the pt. know that you appreciate his efforts to speak; praise & encourage him but remain honest; progress in recalling premorbid language skills is slow & inconsistent;
- be aware that a pt.'s automatic speech may cause you to overestimate his language skills; counting, naming days of week, answering familiar questions with "yes" or "no," & swearing are all forms of automatic speech; to help the pt. progress to effective communication in unfamiliar situations, ask him to identify objects in his room rather than parts of the body; ask him to follow directions or perform simple tasks (pointing, lifting, or counting objects); give prompt & positive feedback for correct answers;
- assist the pt. to recover memory, writing, reading, & speaking skills by starting a progress diary or notebook record of words the pt. can say, sentences s/he has composed, & progress s/he has made; have pt. read it to you & share his pride & growth in regaining language;
- when you have the pt. read to you, ask him to try to explain its meaning (if s/he cannot, explain it & try simpler material but not children's books); if s/he can explain what s/he has read aloud, ask him to read similar matter silently & explain that.

Discharge Planning and Teaching Objectives/Outcomes

1) (Patient/Family/Significant Other) Knows the type of aphasia patient has and how this affects speech, understanding, and other language skills.
2) Has a list of words that patient can say and know(s) to add new words to it.
3) Has a specific short-term goal with date of completion and knows to work on one goal at a time, adding another after successful attainment.
4) Has a referral to/appointment with speech therapist.

Recommended References

"Aphasia and Endurance: Considerations in the Assessment and Care of the Stroke Patient," by M. Louis and S. Povse. *Nursing Clinics of North America*, June 1980:265–276.

Aphasia and the Family. New York: American Heart Association (44 East 23rd Street, 10010).

Aphasia—Hope Through Research, by Office of Scientific and Health Reports. Bethesda, MD: National Institute of Neurological and Communicative Disorders and Stroke (National Institutes of Health, 20205), November 1979.

"Communicating With Your Aphasic Patients," by S. Jennings. *Journal of Practical Nursing*, April 1981:22–39.

Language Problems After A Stroke: A Guide for Communication, by J. Peterson and A. Olsen. Minneapolis: The American Rehabilitation Foundation (1800 Chicago Avenue, 55404).

"Speaking to the Needs of Your Aphasic Patient," by I. Weinhouse. *Nursing 81*, March 1981:34–36.

Stroke: Why Do They Behave That Way? by R. Fowler and W. Fordyce. New York: American Heart Association (44 East 23rd Street, 10010).

"Understanding Aphasia," by S. Norman and R. Baratz. *American Journal of Nursing*, December 1979:2135–2138.

The Patient with an Appendectomy

Definition: Appendectomy is the removal of an inflamed, infected appendix.

LONG TERM GOAL: The patient will recover from the removal of his appendix free of preventable complications; the patient will return to usual roles in home/job/community after a normal short convalescence.

General Considerations:

— **Incidence and occurrence:** appendicitis may occur in any age group, but is seen most frequently in children and young adults; incidence appears to be decreasing in past 10 years.

— **Signs and symptoms:** anorexia, nausea and vomiting; low grade fever, weakness and lethargy; moderate leukocytosis (7,000–17,000/mm); peri-umbilical abdominal tenderness, cramping and pain, shifting after six to 12 hours to the right lower quadrant, localizing at McBurney's point; and rebound tenderness indicating peritoneal irritation.

— **Treatment:** an emergency exploratory laparotomy to remove appendix before rupture; if perforated, drainage with Penrose drains and tubes. Postoperatively, an NG tube remains in place to remove gas and fluid until bowel sounds are heard; then the patient resumes diet and ambulation as tolerated. Morbidity from operating on uncomplicated appendicitis is very low. Complications (abscess, perforation, peritonitis) are much more likely (60%–90%) in patients over 40 and in those whose symptoms last over 36 hours.

— **Preoperative nursing responsibility** is that for general abdominal surgery with the exception of laxatives and enemas, which are not ordered. An NG tube is introduced (refer to NCPG #5:46, "Nasogastric Intubation: General Principles") and dextrose/saline IV infusions are started (refer to NCPG #2:46, "Intravenous Therapy: General Principles"). Parenteral antibiotics are given prophylactically. Studies show that a single dose of metronidazole per intrarectal suppository given 1 hour preoperatively, effectively reduces postoperative wound infection (see Recommended References). Refer to NCPG #2:44, "General Pre-op Care."

— **Postoperative nursing responsibility** is similar to those for general abdominal surgery referred to in NCPGs #2:41–43, "General Post-op Care, Parts A, B, and C."

Specific Considerations, Potential Patient Outcomes, and Nursing Actions:

1) Pulmonary Function — The patient will maintain adequate ventilation; the patient will cough up bronchial secretions; the patient will have clear lungs and be free of atelectasis and pneumonia:

— refer to NCPG #2:41, Part A, "Support of Pulmonary Functions;"
— turn, cough, & deep breathe Q2H;
— monitor & record TPR, noting quality & changes;
— have pt. sit up in high-Fowler's (to facilitate thoracic expansion) as soon as condition permits; leg dangling & progressive ambulation should be done as soon as MD orders.

2) Fluid and Electrolyte Balance

The patient will maintain an optimum fluid and electrolyte balance; the patient will be free of preventable complications:
— accurately monitor & record all fluid intake & output, carefully measuring solution used to irrigate NG tube; estimate diaphoresis & wound drainage;
— palpate suprapubic region for bladder distention; get pt. up to void Q3–4H; if appendix was ruptured & pt. is very sick, a Foley catheter may be used 1st 2 or 3 days;
— administer parenteral fluids, observing administration site for infiltration, redness, leakage;
— refer to NCPG #2:42, Part B, "Support of Cardiovascular Functions;"
— record when peristalsis is heard; know that when intestinal activity is restored, NG tube will be removed; progress pt. from clear liquid diet to soft to regular diet as tolerated.

3) Infection Control

The patient will be free of wound and skin infections:
— note & report temp elevations of 2 or more degrees after the 3rd post-op day;
— administer antibiotics as ordered;
— use strict aseptic technique when changing or handling dressings, drainage tubes, or collection containers.

4) Psychosocial Adjustment and Comfort

The patient will adapt effectively to trauma of surgery and the stress of sudden hospitalization; the patient and family will experience relief of fears and pain and will verbalize feelings of growing strength and independence:
— if perforated, the pt./family will undergo a crisis of serious, life-threatening illness; be as supportive as possible, helping them to sustain each other & be together as much as possible; even if uncomplicated, this is the pt.'s 1st appendectomy & perhaps 1st surgery or hospitalization; the loss of control over one's life is just as important to the pt. as it would be to one of your family;
— administer analgesics liberally 1st 24–48 hours post-op, then PRN, remembering the individual variations of pain thresholds;

- apply ice pack to abdomen PRN if ordered, protecting dressing from moisture;
- apply abdominal binder for support before ambulation, especially if pt. is elderly or overweight;
- as recovery progresses & pt. indicates readiness, begin preparations for discharge with instructions regarding progress, diet, medications, activity, care of incision, & dressing;
- refer to NCPG #2:43, Part C, "Support of Auxiliary Functions."

Discharge Planning and Teaching Objectives/Outcomes:

1) (Patient/Family/Significant Other) Has written appointment, date, and time for follow-up visit to surgeon. Has written instructions regarding activity, diet medications, and care of incision.
2) Knows to call doctor immediately for sudden signs of illness, constipation; pain in abdomen, legs, or chest; increased draining at incision site; or a breaking away of incision.

Recommended References

"General Postoperative Nursing Care, Parts A, B, and C." *NCP Guides #2:41-43*, 2nd Ed., Nurseco, 1980.
"General Preoperative Nursing Care." *NCP Guide #2:44*, 2nd Ed., Nurseco, 1980.
"Intravenous Therapy: General Principles." *NCP Guide #2:46*, 2nd Ed., Nurseco, 1980.
"Management of the Child with Appendicitis," by J. Wakschall. *Journal of Nursing Care*, May 1981:17-21.
"Nasogastric Intubation: General Principles." *NCP Guides #5:46*, Nurseco, 1981.
"Perforated Gangrenous Appendix," by G. Langston. *Nursing Times*, November 20, 1980:2052-2056.
"Single Dose Intrarectal Metronidazole Prophylaxis Against Wound Infection After Appendectomy," by P. Kortelainen et al. *American Journal of Surgery*, February 1982:244-245.
"What Points to Appendicitis?" *Emergency Medicine*, March 15, 1981:47, 49.

The Patient Undergoing Cardiac Catheterization

Definition: A procedure in which a catheter is placed in the heart chambers to determine the functioning and condition of the heart and arteries.

LONG TERM GOAL: The patient will experience a successful cardiac catheterization with minimal anxiety and will be free of preventable complications.

General Considerations:

— The **purpose** of cardiac catheterization is to obtain intracardiac pressure measurements, to obtain blood samples for determination of oxygen content in the various chambers, and to inject radiopaque dyes for determination of presence and location of cardiac and arterial lesions and abnormalities.

— The **site of entry of the catheter** depends on the area of the heart to be studied; femoral and brachial areas are the most common. In left-heart catheterization, the catheter is inserted into an artery and then advanced to the aorta and left heart; in right-heart catheterization, the catheter is inserted into a vein and then advanced to the vena cava and the right heart. The nurse must have information regarding which site is to be used before she orients the patient.

— The injection of the iodine-derivative, radiopaque dye may cause allergic reactions in some patients. Patients should be questioned regarding allergies to iodine and seafood; skin tests are often done to determine any potential reactions to the medium.

— **Potential complications** associated with the procedure are dysrhythmias due to stimulation by the catheter; bleeding at the site of entry; cardiac perforation; myocardial infarction; allergic response to the dye; puncture of a thin-walled vessel; vessel thrombosis; and embolism.

— **Nursing responsibilities** include patient teaching and family counseling regarding reasons for procedure and steps involved, as well as close monitoring of patient for signs of problems during and after procedure.

Specific Considerations, Potential Patient Outcomes, and Nursing Actions:

1) Precatheterization Anxiety and Knowledge of Procedure	The patient will experience no more than a moderate amount of anxiety; the patient will discuss the procedure and verbalize feelings regarding the technique, equipment used, potential risks, side effects of dye and drugs, and postcatheterization period and care: — assess what pt. knows about normal cardiac anatomy & physiology & the planned procedure; encourage questions;

— orient pt. as to what occurs before, during, & after the procedure & why; explain appearance of cath. lab, its equipment, & role of personnel (arrange for a visit to cath. lab if possible);
— ask pt. to share any fears or anxieties with you; share with pt. that other pts. feel as s/he does; know that providing information is one way to reduce fear & anxiety;
— explain to pt. that during the procedure s/he will be strapped (for safety) to an x-ray table, & that the table will be tilted to change position during the examination; that ECG leads will be attached to his extremities; & that s/he will be awake & expected to cooperate with the MD when asked to cough, deep breathe, or hold breath (have pt. practice these procedures);
— prepare pt. for the different sensations s/he will feel during the insertion of the catheter & the injection of the dye (hot, flushed sensation, nausea, palpitations, minimum discomfort in the affected extremity when dye is injected);
— ensure that pt. has been advised of potential risks involved in the procedure & that a written consent has been obtained;
— obtain vital signs to be used as baseline data (apical heart rate, temperature, supine blood pressure, peripheral pulse quality); obtain serum K level to evaluate a potential cause of dysrhythmia;
— have pt. take nothing PO for 6–8 hours prior to the procedure to prevent vomiting & aspiration & to ensure a low BMR during the procedure; ask pt. to void prior to leaving for the lab;
— if pt. is a child, give information according to age (over-preparation for very young children may be upsetting to them); assess what child knows/thinks about procedure; try to liken explanation to what is already familiar to child (e.g., what s/he saw on TV); answer questions & maintain trust; prepare parents as you would an adult pt., to reduce anxiety they might communicate to the child.

2) Postcatheterization Care and Prevention of Complications

The patient will recover from the procedure free of preventable complications:
— assist pt. from the stretcher to the bed; explain that s/he must lie flat with little activity as ordered by the MD (usually 3–6 hours; may be longer if the femoral site was used);
— tell pt. to maintain extension of the extremity used for insertion in order to avoid an increase of pressure in it; advise pt. to report any numbness or pain in the extremity or bleeding at the site;
— check vital signs (including apical pulse) Q15 minutes x 2H, Q30 minutes x 2H, & then Q1H; record all data & report any abnormalities; record I&O for 24 hours;

— inspect pressure dressing on insertion site for bleeding Q15 minutes x 2H; use sandbags for extra pressure PRN;
— check pulses in the extremity distal to insertion site Q15 minutes x 2H; note & report any diminishing of pulse (which may indicate arterial obstruction); check extremity for pallor, cyanosis, lowered temperature, & feelings of tingling & numbness;
— maintain a restful environment as the pt. is usually extremely fatigued due to anxiety & length of procedure.

Discharge Planning and Teaching Objectives/Outcomes

1) (Patient/Family/Significant Other) Knows how to care for catheter injection site.
2) Has follow-up appointment with clinic/doctor.

Recommended References

"A Child's Cardiac Catheterization: Avoiding the Potential Risks," by K. Uzark. *MCN: The American Journal of Maternal Child Nursing*, May/June 1978:158–161.
"Caring for Cardiac Catheterization Patients," by A. Strong. *Nursing 77*, November 1977:60–64.
"Don't Let Cardiac Catheterization Strike Fear in Your Patient's Heart," by D. Teasley. *Nursing 82*, March 1982:52–55.
"Preventing Complications During Cardiac Catheterization," by R. Cogen. *American Journal of Nursing*, March 1976:401–405.
"Reducing Stress in Patients Having Cardiac Catheterization," by C. Finesilver. *American Journal of Nursing*, October 1980:1805–1807.
"Right Heart Catheterization for Intracardiac Electrophysiologic Studies: Implications for the Primary Care Nurse," by C. Gilbert. *Heart and Lung*, January/February 1980:85–92.

The Patient Undergoing Cardiac Surgery (Preoperative Phase)

LONG TERM GOAL: The patient will express adequate knowledge of the existing pathologic condition, technique of correction, and pre- and postoperative care; the patient will be in a stabilized physiologic and psychologic state prior to surgery, and exhibit only moderate anxiety regarding it.

General Considerations:

— **Purpose** of surgery is to correct congenital heart defects, valvular defects, or to revascularize the myocardium in coronary artery disease.

— The **most common type** of myocardial revascularization is the bypass technique, which substitutes an autogenous saphenous vein graft for an obstructed coronary artery by connecting the aorta to the affected artery below the point of atherosclerotic obstruction.

— Myocardial revascularization will correct the existing atherosclerotic ischemic condition, but does not alter the mechanism causing the atherosclerosis; therefore, it is important to educate the patient regarding this and assist him to adapt to the prescribed medical regimen.

— **Contraindications** for myocardial revascularization include severe pump failure with no angina, recent MI with persistent ischemic pain, severe noncardiac disease, and severe anxiety. Controversy exists also as to its benefit in single-vessel disease. Patients with accessible blockage in only one or two vessels may be candidates for percutaneous transluminal coronary angioplasty (PTCA)—inflating a balloon inside a coronary artery to compress an arterial plaque and thereby open the obstructed vessel.

— A thorough diagnostic workup prior to surgery, including cardiac catheterization, ECG, blood coagulation studies, electrolyte and blood gases profile, and circulation time to determine the patient's present status and to be used as baseline information in the postoperative period.

— To diminish probability of complications, the patient should be physiologically and psychologically stable prior to undergoing surgery, i.e., dysrhythmias controlled, weight within acceptable limits, not smoking, free of infection, good pulmonary function, anxiety controlled.

— **Nursing responsibilities** include assessing patient's knowledge and health teaching as needed; preparing patient for postoperative care; and helping patient experience only a moderate degree of preoperative anxiety.

Specific Considerations, Potential Patient Outcomes, and Nursing Actions:

1) Pre-op Teaching

The patient will exhibit no more than moderate anxiety and will be able to discuss important aspects of his diagnosis, surgical correction, and care:

— ask pt. what s/he knows & understands about cardiac pathology, its correction, & the heart-lung machine; provide as much information as s/he wants; do not overburden with information since this may only increase anxiety;
— encourage pt. to verbalize fears, anxieties regarding surgery & to ask questions;
— give pt. general, practical information in which s/he is interested, e.g., visiting hours, length of stay in ICU, availability of chaplain, etc.;
— orient pt. to the pre-op routines & procedures;
— orient pt. to the ICU environment (may be done with pictures or a visit to the ICU), staff, procedures that will be carried out, equipment that may be utilized (endotracheal tube, blow bottles, controlled-volume respirators, IPPB machine, monitoring devices, chest drainage, arterial & venous lines, etc.), & types of sounds normally heard in the ICU (swooshing of respirator, beeps of monitoring equipment);
— explain use of the IPPB apparatus &/or blow bottles, how to do extremity exercises, & the proper techniques of coughing & deep breathing using a pillow on the chest as a splint to reduce pain during coughing; have pt. practice these procedures;
— explain to pt. that because of anxiety, medications, major surgery, the lack of uninterrupted sleep, etc., it is normal to have odd dreams or nightmares, feel depressed, exhausted, or irritable, & that these will pass;
— assure pt. that a nurse will be with him at all times in the ICU & that staff members will be monitoring him closely.

2) Baseline Assessment

The patient's vital signs and psychological status will be recorded for postoperative comparison:

— monitor & record BP, temp, apical & peripheral pulses, weight;
— observe & evaluate psychologic & sociologic behavior of pt. & coping responses; chart level of anxiety (mild, moderate, severe); be aware that severe anxiety may result in post-op delirium & is associated with greater morbidity; investigate the possibility of limited psychotherapeutic intervention if pt. is a poor psychologic risk;
— after health teaching has been done, assess & chart pt.'s expectations regarding post-op pain, results, etc.; are they realistic? unrealistic? correct misconceptions.

3) Pre-op Physical Preparation	The patient will achieve and maintain a stable physical condition in order to diminish the probability of postoperative complications: — have the pt. take Dial or Phisohex showers twice a day for 2–3 days prior to surgery or as ordered by MD; — administer antibiotics prophylactically as ordered, or if pt. has any active infection, including dental infections; — do not permit pt. to smoke for 3–4 days prior to surgery (some MDs may not perform the surgery unless the pt. has agreed to stop smoking); — carry out weight control & dietary measures (low calorie, low cholesterol, low Na) as prescribed by the MD; — administer any meds for control of dysrhythmias, pain, or congestive heart failure; — carry out all routine pre-op orders (NPO, rectal suppository or enema, Foley catheter insertion, skin preparation, & medications).

Discharge Planning and Teaching Objectives/Outcomes

Refer to this section in NCPG #4:07, "The Patient Undergoing Cardiac Surgery: Postoperative Phase."

Recommended References

Refer to this section in NCPG #4:07, "The Patient Undergoing Cardiac Surgery: Postoperative Phase."

The Patient Undergoing Cardiac Surgery (Postoperative Phase)

LONG TERM GOAL: The patient will recover free of preventable complications and return to usual home/job roles while adhering to the prescribed medical regimen.

General Considerations:

— Read this section in NCPG #4:06, "Cardiac Surgery: Preoperative Phase."

— **Nursing responsibilities**, immediately postoperatively, include monitoring the patient for early signs of complications due to the surgery or the patient's basic disease process; taking steps to prevent them; and maintaining the patient in stabilized physiological and psychological states. During later stage of convalescence, nurses are responsible for helping the patient/family prepare for discharge and adjust to medical regimen. Refer to NCPG #4:43, "Diet: Fat-Controlled, Low Cholesterol."

Specific Considerations, Potential Patient Outcomes, and Nursing Actions:

1) Cardiovascular System Assessment and Care

The patient will have normal heart rhythm and will maintain adequate blood volume and fluid and electrolyte balance:

— assess all measurements & observations in relation to pre-op baseline data;

— observe the cardiac monitor for any signs of dysrhythmias; obtain a printout of any abnormalities observed; follow unit protocol for treatment;

— observe & record intra-arterial or cuff BP (intra-arterial pressure is more accurate & may be 10–30 mm Hg higher); be aware that a lowering of diastolic pressure in a pt. with *valve replacement* may be indicative of slippage of the valve resulting in aortic insufficiency; observe carefully & report to MD any signs of hypertension in a pt. with a *bypass* since this could lead to rupture of the graft; be aware of any specific systolic & diastolic limits that may be defined by MD for this pt.;

— assess quality & rate of apical & peripheral pulses, color & warmth of the skin (in order to detect thrombi & emboli);

— when a balloon-tipped, flow-directed catheter (e.g., a Swan-Ganz) is in place, measure pulmonary artery pressure (PAP) & pulmonary wedge pressure (PWP) according to unit protocol; remember that placement of this catheter in the pulmonary artery reflects the functioning of the right heart (the balloon is inflated with room air or carbon dioxide & the catheter advanced (usually by an MD) so that the tip is wedged in a branch of the pulmonary artery; thus the tip is "sealed off" from the right side of the heart & measures the pressure reflected from the left ventricle); *deflate balloon immediately* after taking reading to prevent ischemic damage to the lung & vessel wall due to blockage of blood flow; assess CVP findings in relation to other observations & measurements (ECG, BP, heart sounds, respiration); maintain catheter patency;

— maintain an accurate I&O record to ensure adequate fluid replacement & kidney function; administer fluids as ordered; replace blood lost from chest tube with either blood or fluid as ordered; ask MD for blood loss limits & report excess blood loss immediately; assess quantity & character of urinary output QH; report to MD if urinary output is 25 ml or less/hour for 2 hours; observe pt. for signs of dehydration & overhydration (see NCPGs #3:48 & 49, "Fluids & Electrolytes");

— assist in the monitoring of blood gases, pH, & electrolytes; be aware of pt.'s blood level of K (which might affect cardiac rhythm), & of Na & Cl (which assist in the determination of the hydration status of the pt.); maintain normal serum levels of electrolytes by replacement as ordered by MD (see NCPG #2:48, "Potassium Imbalance").

2) Respiratory System Assessment and Care

The patient will maintain effective normal respirations:

— maintain pt. intubated & on respirator until s/he is able to resume own respiratory functioning & blood gases indicate proper ventilation; be aware of any blood-gas limits that may be defined by MD (endotracheal tube is usually removed after the pt. recovers from anesthesia, which may be as soon as several hours after surgery);

— assess quality & rate of respirations; listen for lung sounds (whether pt. is intubated or not); report diminished breath sounds, rales, or rhonchi; if pt. is intubated, check breath sounds in both lungs & symmetry of breathing to determine if tube has been displaced & slipped into the right mainstem bronchus; observe for congestion in lungs in pts. receiving O_2 by mask attached to a Puritan mist or other aerosol;

— assist pt. with use of IPPB apparatus &/or blow bottles;

— help pt. cough & do deep abdominal breathing Q2H; splint incision with pillow while pt. is coughing; utilize cupping & vibration techniques to loosen secretions; evaluate effectiveness of coughing with chest auscultation; try to arrange giving pain med ½ hour before doing this;

— turn pt. Q2H to prevent atelectasis & retention of secretions;

— suction pt. QH PRN using sterile technique; discard the catheter after each use; ensure that pt. is well oxygenated before, during, & after tracheal suctioning since suctioning decreases the effective tidal volume; apply negative pressure of suction only after catheter is inserted & only for short periods (10–15 seconds) in-

termittently to decrease loss of O_2 & trauma to mucosa; monitor pt.'s ECG carefully during suctioning for any signs of dysrhythmia or ectopic beats; administer O_2 between suctionings to stabilize pt.;
— check patency & drainage of chest tubes; "milk" or "strip" the tubes frequently & regularly to maintain patency & facilitate removal of clots (see NCPG #1:34, "Chest Tubes & Bottles"); notify MD if drainage is more than 100 cc/4H.

3) Pain Relief

The patient will be comfortable and as pain-free as possible:
— observe pt. for nonverbal signs of pain (anxiety, irritability, impaired sleep, crying, facial expressions, restlessness, increased pulse rate);
— encourage pt. to report type, location, & intensity of pain; distinguish between incisional & anginal pain;
— adequately control pain PRN as ordered to make pt. comfortable & to reduce anxiety.

4) Psychologic Support

The patient will experience minimal postoperative anxiety and psychologic reactions:
— explain all new procedures;
— observe pt. for signs of restlessness, disorientation, poor sensory discrimination, or delusions (which may indicate psychologic reactions, lack of sleep, or cerebral ischemia);
— ask pt. directly about any sensory/perceptual difficulties or disturbances s/he may be experiencing; remind pt. of pre-op teaching regarding feelings of depression, irritability, bad dreams, etc.; reassure that these are normal & will pass; be aware that the most common time for these to occur is the 5th–7th day post-op;
— share with pt. any signs or indications of satisfactory progress;
— utilize reorientation techniques with pt. to keep him aware of date, time, place, physical status (open blinds in the morning, call by name, tell date & time, talk about current events);
— encourage visits by the family; share pt.'s status/progress with them; encourage family to touch pt. (arm, face) during visits since touching is more important & effective than talking;
— plan periods of sleep & rest into daily activities; be aware that unfamiliar sounds, monitoring, & pain lead to disturbed sleep, which produces disorientation, anxiety, & depression.

5) Prevention of Complications

The patient will be free of preventable complications and have a normal postoperative convalescence:
— calculate & administer all drugs carefully & specifically, following unit protocol;
— observe wound site for abnormalities;
— maintain strict aseptic technique with chest tubes & urinary drainage;

— assist pt. to perform arm & shoulder exercises ("climbing the wall," hands on shoulders with elbows circling) to prevent stiffness & immobility;
— plan progressive ambulation & activity with periods of rest, according to the individual's capabilities & type of surgery performed.

Discharge Planning and Teaching Objectives/Outcomes

1) (Patient/Family/Significant Other) Can discuss the desirability of maintaining normal weight and the diet s/he is to follow at home.
2) Demonstrates an understanding of the progressive exercise regimen, the desirability of daily walks except in cold weather, and the importance of not lifting heavy objects (10–15 lb limit for four weeks since heavy lifting causes stress on incision and a rise in intrathoracic pressure).
3) Will incorporate rest periods into progressive daily activities and will rest when tired.
4) Can identify medications, their purposes and side effects, and verbalizes the importance of taking the prescribed dosage at the prescribed times.
5) Will avoid activities and habits considered to be risk factors.
6) Will seek adequate medical supervision during convalescent period and can identify factors that necessitate a call to the physician postoperatively.
7) Knows date and time of first follow-up office visit.

Recommended References

"Central Venous Pressure Line." *NCP Guide #2:40*, 2nd Ed., Nurseco, 1980.
"Chest Tubes and Bottles: Water-seal Drainage." *NCP Guide #1:34*, 2nd Ed., Nurseco, 1980.
"Diet: Fat-Controlled, Low Cholesterol." *NCP Guide #4:43*, 2nd Ed., Nurseco, 1983.
"Exciting New Alternatives to Coronary By-pass Surgery," by R. Sprengel. *RN*, December 1981:24–27.
"Fluids and Electrolytes." *NCP Guides #3:48, 49*, 2nd Ed., Nurseco, 1983.
"How Open Heart Surgery Feels," by H. Derrick. *American Journal of Nursing*, February 1979:277–285.
"Intracoronary Streptokinase Infusion," by L. Wadsworth et al. *Nursing 82*, May 1982:58–65.
"Nursing Assessment of Postcardiotomy Delirium," by P. Sadler. *Heart and Lung*, July/August 1978:987–994.
"A Nursing Care Plan—The Adult Cardiac Surgery Patient," by C. Thorpe. *Heart and Lung*, July/August 1979:690–698.
"Phases of Recovery from Open-Heart Surgery," by C. Jillings. *Heart and Lung*, November/December 1978:987–994.
"Potassium Imbalance." *NCP Guide #2:48*, 2nd Ed., Nurseco 1980.
"This Procedure Called PTCA: Your Patient's CABG Substitute?" by K. Scordo. *Nursing 82*, February 1982:50–55.
"What Open-Heart Surgery Patients Want to Know," by R. Mayer et al. *American Journal of Nursing*, September 1979:1558–1560.

The Patient in Cardiogenic Shock

Definition: An acute state of decreased cardiac output and decreased tissue perfusion caused by left ventricular pump failure.

LONG TERM GOAL: The patient will regain optimum perfusion of vital organs with gradual withdrawal of supportive measures through correction of underlying cause and improvement of cardiovascular action.

General Considerations:

— **Incidence:** may occur in patients with severe congestive heart failure, cor pulmonale, myocardial pericarditis, and in 15%-20% of patients with acute myocardial infarction.

— **Mortality rate** of cardiogenic shock persisting more than one hour is about 80%. Therefore, early detection and correction of impending shock is crucial.

— **Signs and symptoms** include evidence of cerebral hypoxia (confusion, restlessness, apathy), tachycardia, peripheral vasoconstriction (skin cold, profuse sweating, pallor), decreased or absent peripheral pulses (result of hypoperfusion), decreased urinary output (less than 20 ml/hour), decreased blood pressure (systolic below 80 mm Hg or more than 30 mm Hg below patient's "normal" systolic pressure) with narrowing of pulse pressure, and increased respirations with short, shallow respiratory efforts.

— **Treatment** is aimed at improving cardiovascular function through supportive measures such as sympathomimetics and mechanical ventilation. If improvement does not occur, an intra-aortic balloon pump may be inserted to reduce left ventricular filling pressure and improve output and flow. If these are not effective, the patient may be prepared for cardiac catheterization and possible open heart surgery to correct the cause of the cardiovascular failure.

— **Nursing responsibilities** include closely observing patient for signs of impending cardiogenic shock and carrying out emergency treatment measures.

Specific Considerations, Potential Patient Outcomes, and Nursing Actions:

1) Restoration/ Maintenance of Tissue Perfusion and Intravascular Volume	The patient will regain proper perfusion of vital organs through improved cardiac action: — administer O_2 at high flow; an endotracheal tube may be inserted & pt. placed on a volume-cycled ventilator; — administer & observe proper flow of IVs used to maintain effective circulating volume (DW, Dextran, albumin); — administer antidysrhythmic & vasopressor agents as prescribed by MD; be aware that some MDs now use vasodilating drugs in conjunction with adequate fluid volume replacement; calculate & administer all drugs carefully & specifically; utilize metriset or similar equipment for controlling volume & rapidity of IV drugs.

2) Prevention of Complications

The patient will be free of preventable complications; the patient will be monitored closely for early signs of potential complications:

— insert Foley catheter & record urinary output QH; remember that an increase in the quantity of urine produced is a sign of increased tissue perfusion; measure specific gravity of the urine to determine its concentration; keep an accurate I&O; assess insensible fluid loss (through perspiration, lungs, & suctioning);

— monitor cuff or intra-arterial blood pressure Q5–15 minutes to determine changes in systolic pressure & pulse pressure; monitor rate, quality, & rhythm of pulse;

— if a CVP line in place, measure CVP, which reflects right cardiac functioning, vascular tone, & circulating blood volume; ensure that the catheter is properly placed in the superior vena cava & that it is maintained at a consistent zero-level at the level of the right atrium approximately half way between the anterior & posterior chest wall; mark the baseline zero-level on the pt.'s chest; see NCPG #2:40, "Central Venous Pressure Line;"

— when a balloon-tipped, flow-directed catheter (e.g., a Swan-Ganz) is in place, measure pulmonary artery pressure (PAP) & pulmonary wedge pressure (PWP) according to unit protocol; remember that placement of this catheter in the pulmonary artery reflects the functioning of the right heart (the balloon is inflated with room air or CO_2 & the catheter advanced (usually by an MD) so that the tip is wedged in a branch of the pulmonary artery; thus the tip is "sealed off" from the right side of the heart & measures the pressure reflected from the left ventricle); *deflate balloon immediately* after taking reading to prevent ischemic damage to the lung & vessel wall due to blockage of blood flow; maintain catheter patency;

— be aware that CVP, PAP, & PWP monitoring are guides to the adequacy of fluid replacement & drug therapy; remember that vasopressors & other hemodynamic drugs are not given via these lines as they would enter the heart very rapidly in concentrated form;

— monitor ECG readings to determine the presence of dysrhythmias, which can be rapidly fatal if not diagnosed promptly; recognize that dysrhythmias may be present following an MI or as a result of metabolic disorders leading to hypoxia, acidosis, hypokalemia, or hyperkalemia; see NCPG #3:40, "Acid-Base Balance;"

— assess effectiveness of counterpulsation techniques, if used, such as external counterpulsation or the intra-aortic balloon pumping device; monitor leg perfusion since balloon may result in decreased vascular perfusion in leg with cutdown; check leg for temperature & pulse changes;

- — monitor blood gases & pH; be aware of pt.'s blood levels of K (which can affect cardiac rhythm) & of Na & Cl (which assist in the determination of the hydration status); see NCPG #2:48, "Potassium Imbalance;"
- — assess pt.'s level of consciousness frequently;
- — maintain strict aseptic technique especially at invasive-line sites, since pt.'s immunological response is decreased during shock; cleanse sites daily with acetone & Betadine & cover with a sterile, occlusive dressing (check for allergic reaction to iodine before using Betadine); wear mask & sterile gloves for these dressing changes;
- — report & record any observed changes in pt.'s status.

3) Rest and Comfort

The patient will be comfortable and experience reduced or controlled pain:

- — conserve pt.'s energy at onset; place pt. in semi-Fowler's position; do not move pt. unnecessarily; carry out only the most essential care measures;
- — administer analgesics as prescribed for pain & discomfort;
- — suction PRN; turn from side to side; use cupping & vibration techniques to prevent atelectasis.

4) Anxiety and Fear

The patient will be oriented to the situation and will establish a means of communicating needs and concerns; the patient will experience and express no more than moderate fear and anxiety:

- — recognize that the pt. may be aware of the situation & experience feelings of helplessness & fright during this period, even though his level of consciousness may be diminished; acknowledge these feelings; share with pt. any signs of positive change;
- — orient the pt. to what you are doing & why;
- — carry out procedures with confidence & efficiency to make the pt. feel more secure;
- — utilize touch & supportive words to ease anxiety;
- — set up nonverbal means of communication for pt. who is intubated or too weak to talk, but conscious enough to make needs known;
- — utilize personnel skilled in crisis intervention, if available, to assist the family & give them emotional support.

Recommended References

"Acid-Base Balance." *NCP Guide #3:40*, 2nd Ed., Nurseco, 1983.
"Cardiac Emergency! How to Use Drugs & CPR to Save Lives," by C. Ciaverelli Manzi. *Nursing 78*, March 1978:30-39.
"Cardiogenic Shock: Catch It Early!" by C. Crumlish. *Nursing 81*, August 1981:34-41.
"Central Venous Pressure Line." *NCP Guide #2:40*, 2nd Ed., Nurseco, 1980.
Comprehensive Cardiac Care, 4th Ed., by K. Andreoli et al. St. Louis: Mosby, 1979.
"Fluids & Electrolytes." *NCP Guides #3:48, 49*, 2nd Ed., Nurseco, 1983.
"Intraortic Balloon Pumping: Concepts and Patient Care," by A. Chrzanowski. *Nursing Clinics of North America*, September 1978: 513-530.
"Potassium Imbalance." *NCP Guide #2:48*, 2nd Ed., Nurseco, 1980.
"Shock Demands Drugs—But Which One's Best for Your Patient?" by J. Barrows. *Nursing 82*, February 1982:34-41.

The Patient with a Cerebral Aneurysm

Definition: A dilated (outpouched) area of an intracranial arterial wall that is weakened and susceptible to leakage or rupture.

LONG TERM GOAL: The patient will have neurological condition stabilized in preparation for surgical intervention to repair aneurysm and traumatic results of its leakage or rupture. If inoperable because of critical condition, the patient will be sustained for as long as possible and the patient and family will be helped to cope with the crisis of loss.

General Considerations:

— **Incidence:** aneurysmal subarachnoid hemorrhage strikes an estimated 11 per 1000 population.

— **Signs and symptoms** vary according to patient and amount of bleeding (subarachnoid hemorrhage). Unruptured intracranial aneurysms are often asymptomatic. A five-grade system is used to categorize levels of severity:
Grade 1: alert, no neurological deficit, minimal headache, and minimal nuchal (neck) rigidity
Grade 2: mild to severe headache and nuchal rigidity, neurological deficit related to 3rd cranial nerve palsy (drooping eyelid, diplopia, unilateral pupil dilation or visual loss due to compression of optic chiasm)
Grade 3: drowsy, confused, mild deficit
Grade 4: stupor, mild to severe hemiparesis
Grade 5: deep coma, decerebrate rigid extension, moribund appearance.
Other symptoms that may be associated with a leaking aneurysm are nausea, vomiting, loss of consciousness and/or orientation, neck and back pain, and photophobia. Vital signs are normal if bleeding is minimal, but body temperature becomes elevated as blood increases in the CSF. Hypertension is present in more than half of cases. Stress (physical and emotional) is often associated with precipitation of aneurysmal rupture.

— **Diagnosis** is made with a thorough neurological exam followed by lumbar puncture revealing increased intracranial pressure (ICP) and bloody spinal fluid. CT brain scans and cerebral angiography are used to locate the lesion. Refer to NCPG #5:04, "The Patient Needing Angiography."

— **Prognosis:** about nine out of 10 patients are not diagnosed until after aneurysm has ruptured and subarachnoid hemorrhage has occurred. Approximately 30%–50% die immediately; another 20% who survive the initial hemorrhage succumb from rebleeding, vasospasm, ischemia, and/or cerebral edema in the first 10 days.

— **Treatment** aims to save the patient's life, maintain and stabilize his condition during the first critical phase, prevent rebleeding, keep the intracranial pressure at safe levels, and prepare for surgery. Surgery involves clipping, ligating, or wrapping the aneurysm. Patients able to undergo surgical repair of the aneurysm usually recover with few complications and mild neurological deficits. Patients who are poor surgical risks because of age, debility, other diseases, etc., are treated conservatively with two to four weeks of bedrest, hypotensive medications (when indicated), ICP control measures, and Amicar (inhibits fibrinolysis and strengthens the aneurysm seal thereby reducing or preventing recurrent hemorrhage).

— **Nursing responsibilities** include

1) sharing with the patient/family/significant other the possibility of death and encouraging them to express their fears and feelings; provide crisis intervention as needed (refer to NCPG #2:30, "The Patient Needing Crisis Intervention");
2) providing life-support measures aimed at meeting treatment goals and enlisting the aid of the family in establishing an optimal therapeutic environment for the patient (If the patient is to be saved, intensive primary (one on one) nursing care is needed); and
3) writing a detailed referral for home health nurse or convalescent hospital staff giving neurological deficits and physical limitations, emotional and mental status assessment, plan for rehabilitation and the involvement of the family.

Specific Considerations, Potential Patient Outcomes, and Nursing Actions:

1) Control of Hemorrhage and Prevention of Complications

The patient will maintain optimal conditions to reduce threat of rebleeding, cerebral vasospasm, decreased perfusion, ischemia, infarction, and edema; the patient will maintain a safe level of intracranial pressure:

— know that pt. is often admitted to a neurological ICU attended by clinical specialists; otherwise provide complete bed rest in a darkened, quiet, private room;

— elevate head of bed 20°–30°;

— do not permit TV, but soft, soothing music known to be liked by pt. or relaxation tapes may prove helpful & therapeutic; limit visitors to 1 member of family or close friend at a time & only for 15–30 minutes/visit; permit some flexibility if pt. is deteriorating & not expected to survive;

— monitor vital signs, CVP, & ICP carefully & accurately;

— encourage periods of undisturbed sleep or rest but avoid clustering several nursing activities that will increase ICP (e.g., suctioning, drawing blood gases, bathing pt.); turn pt. slowly, gently, & with assistance; postpone unnecessary bed linen changes; transport pt. smoothly & unhurriedly;

— give stool softeners to prevent straining at defecation; avoid harsh laxatives or cathartics, suppositories, enemas, or rectal temps; stay with pt. while on bedpan;

— give antiemetics for nausea to prevent vomiting (which will increase ICP & may disturb clot);

- — employ seizure precautions (padded bedrails, tongue blade, & endotracheal tube at bedside) but avoid wrist & ankle restraints (which often produce restlessness & upset pt.);
- — provide only passive range-of-motion exercises; do not permit isometric exercises, pushing against footboard, or breathholding while being moved (they increase ICP);
- — give hypotensive agents as ordered & check vital signs QH, reporting sudden or progressive changes;
- — take care to record I&O *accurately* (an important record to watch); restrict fluids & give IV fluids with a microdrip chamber;
- — if conscious, feed liquids slowly; if unconscious, pass NG tube & attach to intermittent suction; if pt. is on steroids to control cerebral edema, give with milk & antacids;
- — observe & assess neurological status; refer to NCPGs #4:01, "The Patient with an Acute Head Injury," & #4:11, "The Patient with Acutal/Potential IIP;" observe & report signs of possible rebleeding of aneurysm (headache, nausea, lethargy, neck & back pain); observe & report signs of possible ischemia, vasospasm, or occlusion at site of aneurysm (motor or sensory impairment of extremities);
- — if administering epsilon-aminocaproic acid (EACA, Amicar), know that bradycardia, dysrhythmias, & hypotension have been seen after rapid IV administration; if given orally as a tablet or syrup, watch for difficulty swallowing or choking; be alert to untoward reactions (cramping, *diarrhea*, dizziness, nausea, tinnitus, & skin rash); observe for signs of superficial or deep vein thrombosis & pulmonary embolism;
- — to prevent cerebral vasospasm secondary to subarachnoid hemorrhage, be prepared to give, as ordered, Reserpine (usually 0.1 mg QID SQ) and Kanamycin (1 Gm TID *orally*; ineffective on serotonin in GI tract if given IM); know, observe, & record expected side effects of hypotension & diarrhea; know that these drugs are ineffective & thus discontinued once vasospasm has occurred;
- — know that in the event of cerebral vasospasm, expert nursing care is directed toward maintaining cerebral perfusion, keeping the pt.'s BP in a *hyper*tensive state of approximately 140–160 mm Hg; very carefully & accurately monitor vital signs & neurological signs Q15 minutes, fluid & electrolyte infusion speed & volume, & administration of vasopressors, packed red blood cells;
- — keep currently knowledgeable on the rationale for the above critical nursing & medical care measures, since there is still no universally accepted treatment for prevention & treatment of cerebral vasospasm.

2) Maintenance of Vital Functions	The patient will be free of preventable complications, maintaining intact skin, adequate respiratory function, fluid and electrolyte balance, sufficient urinary output: — provide oral hygiene Q4H using lemon-glycerin swabs, mouthwash, Water Pik, or gentle irrigation with syringe; apply lubricant to lips; — remove dried secretions from eyes with cotton pads moistened with normal saline; instill artificial tears (methyl-cellulose drops); keep eyelids closed with pad & tape; — keep skin clean, dry, & as pressure-free as possible; use standard decubitus prevention measures; — use footboards, trochanter rolls, splints, or towel rolls to maintain functional position & prevent contractures; — note urine output QH & report to MD if below 30cc (or 100 cc per voiding); note & record specific gravity & appearance; avoid indwelling catheter if possible but know that urinary retention causes restlessness, retention with overflow, or URI; — explain all actions to pt.; state what is happening & why; answer questions & speak to pt. frequently to allay fears & calm him; provide repeated explanations to family & give them an opportunity to ask questions or express feelings.
3) Pre- & Post-op Nursing Considerations, Outcomes, and Actions	Refer to NCPG #4:12, "The Patient with Intracranial Surgery."

Discharge Planning and Teaching Objectives/Outcomes

1) (Patient/Family/Significant Other) Has received written instructions and verbalizes understanding and acceptance of convalescent status with restrictions. Has received referral phone numbers of home health service, social service disability office, homemaker service, and other appropriate community resources.
2) Knows medications, dosages, indications, and side effects to be reported. Has list of speech, writing, physical exercises to be performed daily.

3) Has written appointment date and time for medical follow-up.
4) Understands that eyelid ptosis may persist indefinitely but need not interfere with getting around or driving; that wearing an eyepatch while driving is recommended because judging distance is lacking in the affected eye.
5) Knows that current problems, if present (residual hemiparesis, memory deficits, dysphasia, visual impairment), should not progressively worsen during convalescent period and, if they do, to seek immediate medical treatment. Knows to see doctor promptly for signs of confusion, headache, nausea, vomiting, fever, or other questionable symptoms.

Recommended References

"A Holding Action In Subarachnoid Hemorrhage." *Emergency Medicine*, April 30, 1981:49, 50.
"Intra-operative Aneurysm Clipping," by D. Morris. *Journal of Neurosurgical Nursing*, June 1982:150–153.
"The Patient with an Acute Head Injury." *NCP Guide #4:01*, 2nd Ed., Nurseco, 1983.
"The Patient with Actual/Potential Increased Intracranial Pressure." *NCPG Guide #4:11*, 2nd Ed., Nurseco, 1983.
"The Patient Needing Angiography." *NCP Guide #5:04*, Nurseco, 1981.
"The Patient Needing Crisis Intervention." *NCP Guide #2:31*, 2nd Ed., Nurseco, 1980.
"The Patient with Intracranial Surgery." *NCP Guide #4:12*, 2nd Ed., Nurseco, 1983.
"Sending Cerebral Aneurysms to Surgery." *Emergency Medicine*, September 30, 1981:139, 140.
"Treating Subarachnoid Haemorrhage Using Carotid Ligation," by D. Allan. *Nursing Times*, August 5, 1981:1383–1385.
"Vasospasm Secondary to Subarachnoid Hemorrhage: The Current Controversy, Research, and Nursing Dilemmas," by K. Finch. *Journal of Neurosurgical Nursing*, December 1980:199–202.

The Patient with a Herniorrhaphy

Definition: Herniorrhaphy is the surgical repair of an abnormal protrusion of an organ through the muscle wall, which usually contains it.

LONG TERM GOAL: The patient will recover from the repair of a hernia free of preventable complications; the patient will return to usual roles in home/job/community after a normal short convalescence.

General Considerations:

— **Types:** inguinal protrusion is four times more common than other sites: femoral, umbilical, ventral, and incisional. Hernias are called "reducible" if they can be manipulated easily back into place or "irreducible" (also known as "incarcerated") if they cannot. Hernias are deemed "strangulated" if the blood supply has been cut off to the protruding part.

— **Treatment** is aimed at medically reducing the herniated tissue or surgically excising it and repairing the defective wall. The patient without complications is discharged within two to six days. Some patients are now being surgically treated on an outpatient basis under local anesthesia in surgicenters.

— **Nursing responsibilities** are those outlined in NCPGs #2:44, "General Pre-op Care," and #s 2:41–43, "General Post-op Care, Parts A, B, and C." Early ambulation is urged and measures are taken to reduce probabilities of recurrence (see below).

Specific Considerations, Potential Patient Outcomes, and Nursing Actions:

1) Pulmonary Function

The patient will maintain adequate ventilation; the patient will cough up bronchial secretions; the patient will have clear lungs and be free of atelectasis and pneumonia:

— refer to NCPG #2:41, Part A: "Support of Pulmonary Functions;"

— turn, cough, & deep breathe Q2H; IPPB treatments are given to stimulate deep breathing & mucus removal; give pain medication 30 minutes before treatments; cover incision with pillow & hands to support incision before coughing; teach pt. importance of doing this;

— monitor & record TPR, noting quality & changes;

— have pt. sit up in high-Fowler's (to facilitate thoracic expansion) as soon as condition permits; leg dangling & progressive ambulation should be done as soon as MD orders; apply abdominal binder when pt. is up walking; note posture & urge pt. to stand erect to prevent shortening of abdominal muscles & habitual stooping.

2) Fluids and Electrolytes

The patient will maintain an optimum fluid and electrolyte balance and be free of preventable complications:

— accurately monitor & record all I&O, carefully measuring solution used to irrigate NG tube; estimate

diaphoresis & wound drainage;
— palpate suprapubic region for bladder distention; get pt. up to void, if possible, Q3–4H; if Foley catheter in place, keep unkinked & draining well; give routine indwelling catheter care;
— administer parenteral fluids, observing administration site for infiltration, redness, leakage; see NCPG #2:46, "Intravenous Therapy: General Principles;"
— refer to NCPG #2:42, Part B, "Support of Cardiovascular Functions."

3) Infection Control
The patient will be free of wound and skin infections:
— note & report temperature elevations of 2 or more degrees after 3rd post-op day;
— administer antibiotics as ordered;
— use strict aseptic technique when changing or handling dressings.

4) Psychosocial Adjustment and Comfort
The patient will adapt effectively to trauma of surgery and the stress of hospitalization; the patient will verbalize relief from pain and fears and will express a growing confidence with self-care:
— administer analgesics liberally 1st 24–28 hours post-op & after that, when deemed necessary, remembering individual variations in pain threshold;
— be available to pt./family for expression of comments, feelings, & questions;
— as recovery progresses & the pt. indicates readiness, begin preparations for discharge with instructions regarding progress, activity, exercise, medications, & care of incision & dressing.

Discharge Planning and Teaching Objectives/Outcomes

1) (Patient/Family/Significant Other) States s/he knows activity restrictions: (a) lift nothing heavier than a book for four weeks; (b) walk 10–20 minutes twice daily with erect posture; (c) avoid strenuous sports or manual labor for six weeks.
2) Knows how to prevent constipation that would cause unnecessary tension on healing sutures.
3) Has written appointment for follow-up visit to surgeon. Has written instructions for activity limitations and care of incision.
4) Knows to call doctor immediately for sudden signs of illness, pain in abdomen, legs or chest, increasing drainage at incision site, or breaking away of sutures.

Recommended References

"General Postoperative Nursing Care, Parts A, B, and C." *NCP Guides #2:41-43*, 2nd Ed., Nurseco, 1980.
"General Preoperative Nursing Care." *NCP Guide #2:44*, 2nd Ed., Nurseco, 1980.
"Herniorrhaphies Performed Upon Outpatients Under Local Anesthesia," by L. Flanagan and J. Bascom. *Surgery, Gynecology and Obstetrics*, October 1981:557–560.
"Intravenous Therapy: General Principles." *NCP Guide #2:46*, 2nd Ed., Nurseco, 1980.

The Patient with Actual/Potential Increased Intracranial Pressure

Definition: Increased intracranial pressure (IIP) is a rise above normal of the pressure of the cerebrospinal fluid in the subarachnoid space. The normal intracranial pressure (ICP) ranges between 0 and 15 mm Hg.

LONG TERM GOAL: The patient will maintain stable vital functions with minimum complications throughout the period of actual or potential increased intracranial pressure. The patient will experience reduction of increased intracranial pressure with no residual neurological deficits. When possible, the cause of the increased intracranial pressure will be identified and resolved.

General Considerations:

— **Causes:** following a serious head injury, IIP results from cerebral bleeding, nervous-tissue edema, or depressed skull fractures. IIP is also brought about by brain congestion imposed by an infarction or by a space-occupying lesion (neoplasm, hematoma, aneurysm, congenital malformation, or abscess). Generalized brain swelling may also occur as a result of anoxic situations such as drowning, smoke inhalation, asphyxia, accidents, infections, or chemical toxicity.

— **Signs and symptoms:** decreasing level of consciousness (LOC) and lessened responsiveness (decreased motor response to command, decreased sensory response to painful stimuli); pupillary changes (decreased reactivity to light), papilledema (swelling of optic disc), changes in eye movement, diplopia, and decreased vision; reduced strength, movement, and sensitivity of extremities; rising systolic blood pressure and increasing pulse pressure; bradycardia and slowing pulse; increasingly severe headache, persistent nausea and vomiting; rapid, irregular respiration with pauses; loss of bladder or bowel control; seizures; decorticate or decerebrate posturing (see explanation below).

— **Diagnostic measures** include skull films, cervical spine series (to level of C-7, T-1) and computerized tomography (CT) scans. An ICP monitoring device, while still controversial, is commonly used. One method is a Richmond screw placed below the dura into subarachnoid space, connected with tubing to a transducer, producing a readout on a graph. Another method is the insertion of a catheter or cannula into the lateral ventricle (also connected to a transducer).

— **Treatment** to reduce IIP includes

- maintaining adequate ventilation to prevent cerebral hypoxia and hypercarbia (CO_2 is a vasodilator, thereby increasing cerebral blood flow and pressure);
- (if spinal cord injury has been ruled out) elevation of the head of the bed 15°–30° to facilitate venous outflow;

- administration of osmotic diuretics to remove water from intracerebral cells; care must be taken to prevent dehydration, electrolyte imbalance, and rebound effect of prolonged usage;
- administration of steroids to prevent cerebral edema; concurrent administration of antacids to reduce gastric ulceration;
- pharmacologically-induced paralysis of voluntary muscles to prevent ICP spikes caused by physical movements in response to various stimuli;
- hypothermia will occasionally be used to reduce metabolism, body's oxygen requirements, and cerebral blood flow;
- barbiturates QH to maintain a serum level of 3 mg/100 ml blood volume in order to decrease brain metabolism and oxygen demand, therefore blood flow to brain;
- surgical intervention to remove hematoma, aneurysm, or other cause of IIP; surgical decompression measures such as a ventricular drain or a removal of a bone flap to allow for expansion of brain tissue.

— **Nursing responsibilities** include (1) arranging for one-to-one (if possible) primary care in a neurological intensive care unit to provide reliable, consistent, competent neurological observations and assessments; (2) planning, implementing, and evaluating medical therapy and nursing care to prevent and control IIP (a standard protocol developed by your own neurological specialists is most helpful); (3) constantly monitoring measures to maintain vital functions and patient's response to therapy. Be aware of effect of medications, physical movements, or conditions that may affect ICP, mask signs or potentiate them, make interpretation and accurate assessment more difficult; (4) keeping family honestly informed as to patient's progress, prognosis, and plan of treatment; encouraging realistic hope and providing emotional support to facilitate stress management; use crisis intervention applicable.

Specific Considerations, Potential Patient Outcomes, and Nursing Actions:

1) Neurological Observation and Assessment

The patient's neurological status will be continually monitored for changes indicating a need for intervention; early signs of IIP will be identified and reported immediately:

— know clearly the different levels of consciousness (LOC) & *describe* pt. clearly, carefully, & comprehensively:

1) *Full Consciousness*: alert; responsive to auditory, tactile, & visual stimuli; oriented to person, place, & time (PPT); intact memory for recent events; has insight into condition; verbalizes readily, coherently, & distinctly (ask why or when questions rather than those requiring a simple yes or no reply);
2) *Impaired Consciousness/Drowsiness/Lethargy*: loss of recent memory and insight; slower thinking but still rather alert with intelligible & appropriate responses; (report these subtle changes to MD & increase frequency of neuro checks);

3) *Confusion/Delirium*: transient periods of disorientation, restlessness, uncooperativeness; dazed, easily agitated, & irritable when disturbed; fearful, noisy; still responding to verbal stimuli & light tactile stimuli such as pin pricks or a light pinch on the neck;
4) *Stupor*: responds only to repeated insistent verbal stimuli or continuous, painful tactile stimuli such as mandibular, sternal, or periorbital pressure;
5) *Coma*: response to intense stimuli is either reflex or absent; (NOTE: Some neuro units use the Glasgow Coma Scale (GCS) Index—see Recommended References by C. Jones, & Connolly & Zewe—which is becoming more widespread, although a clear behavior description by a reliable observer may be preferred.)

— obtain frequent (Q15 minutes) vital signs & continuing checks of LOC;

— observe & record *pupillary signs*, L&R: size (small, medium, large, or some hospital protocols require measurement of pupil with a metric ruler); equality (remember that about 25% of normal people have *slightly* unequal pupils); reactivity or response to light in a dimly shaded room (record reaction as brisk, sluggish, or nonreactive/fixed & report STAT dilating pupils reacting sluggishly to light);

— check eye movement (up, down, to sides, are eyes moving together? have pt. follow your finger without moving head);

— check upper & lower *extremities* & digits for *strength*, *movement*, & *sensation*; observe for both spontaneous movement & response to simple commands "squeeze my two fingers," "raise your left/right leg," "push against my hand"); use gradually increasing sensory stimuli (gentle stroking → pin prick → deep pressure pain) & record response as *complex* (withdrawal from stimulus & attempt to remove it) or *simple* (only withdrawal from stimulus); note if *posturing* is *decorticate* (rigid flexion of head, arm(s), wrist(s), fingers & plantar flexion with internal rotation of limb(s)) or *decerebrate* (rigid extension of head, neck, back with hyperpronation of limb(s));

— check *vital signs* Q30 minutes (know that changes usually develop *after* LOC diminishes, & that vital sign changes are compensatory in nature); report STAT *bradycardia* & slowly falling pulse rate (taken for 1 minute), followed by a sharply rising pulse rate; *rising systolic pressure* & *widening pulse pressure* (normal difference between systolic & diastolic pressure = 40); *alterations in respiratory rate & rhythm* (describe & report if Cheyne-Stokes type, if hyperventilation, if there are apneustic-sustained pauses, clustered breathing, or ataxic breathing; know that temperature is not valid indicator of IIP (temp may or may not rise; aspirin or acetaminophen given for headache may keep temp near normal);

— provide for ECG monitoring with full alarm system;
— be aware of effect of medications, physical movements, or conditions that may affect ICP, mask signs or potentiate them, or make interpretation and accurate assessment more difficult;
— if ICP monitoring device is in place, arrange for careful, accurate, regular, & continuous measurement of ICP (*especially* in *children* & *aged* who have lower tolerance for intracerebral volume change); check for need to recalibrate or reposition transducer, or flush tubing regularly to ensure accurate readings; know that even the smallest air bubble can cause inaccurate pressure reading; do not allow tubing to be kinked; keep pt.'s head in alignment with body to promote correct functioning;
— know that cerebral perfusion pressure (CPP), the mean arterial pressure minus the mean ICP, must be at least 50 mm Hg to sustain normal cerebral blood flow (the mean arterial pressure (MAP) is calculated by adding the diastolic pressure to 1/3 the pulse pressure.)

2) Maintenance of Vital Functions and Prevention of Complications

The patient's IIP will diminish; the patient will survive without irreversible brain damage; the patient will maintain adequate fluid and electrolyte balance, cardiopulmonary function, and elimination, and be free of infection; the patient's vital signs will stabilize:
— refer to this section in NCPG #4:01, "The Patient with an Acute Head Injury;"
— elevate head of bed 15°–30° to promote cerebral venous drainage by gravity;
— maintain a patent airway to prevent hypoxia & hypercarbia (side-lying position for comatose pts.);
— if pt. has ICP greater than 20 mm Hg for 4 hours or longer, know that pharmacological coma may be therapeutically induced with barbiturates to decrease brain metabolism & O_2 demand, thus reducing cerebral edema by enhancing cerebral vasoconstriction; know that a Swan-Ganz catheter must be inserted (if not already in place) so that intravascular volume can be monitored; since neurological assessment will be extremely difficult, *all* clinical parameters must be closely & continuously monitored with full alarm systems operational; after determining ICP & MAP, calculate cerebral perfusion pressure (MAP minus ICP) & maintain at 60–70 mm Hg; know that barbiturate therapy is tapered off gradually when ICP has been normalized for 72 hours or there is a lack of response to this treatment; know that a slowed reaction time & a lack of facial response for several days is to be expected;
— if administering mannitol (given rapidly as an IV bolus over 10-20 minutes to temporarily relieve cerebral edema) know that a rebound increase in ICP may occur approximately 12 hours later; know that fluid imbalances & renal complications may occur; watch also for side effects of headache, nausea, vomiting, chills,

polydipsia, dizziness, lethargy; watch for angina-like chest pain; report all untoward signs STAT;

— closely monitor arterial blood gases (ABGs) & listen to chest sounds regularly; know that the pCO_2 should be 25–30 mg Hg (never below 20 or above 35); pO_2 should be 70–80 mg Hg higher; suction PRN, but limit to 15 seconds to minimize CO_2 accumulation; keep an Ambu bag attached to 100% oxygen & endotracheal intubation equipment nearby for emergency use; know that pts. with a GCS Index of 8 or less (stuporous, semicomatose) & deteriorating will be intubated & placed on controlled ventilation;

— carefully monitor & accurately record I&O, especially urine output QH, when hyperosmolar diuretics are used; watch for signs of dehydration & hypovolemic shock especially in children & elderly debilitated persons; observe for electrolyte imbalance (behavior changes, muscle weakness, diminished reflexes, changes in urine specific gravity & blood serum values);

— pad side rails & take seizure precautions, especially if pt. has a seizure history, a skull fracture, a GCS score of 8 or less; have diphenylhydantoin (Dilantin) & diazepam (Valium) for parenteral use readily available;

— know, teach, & evaluate the effect of nursing activities on the pt.'s ICP;

— turn pt. slowly & gently; have pt. exhale while turning to prevent Valsalva maneuver (breath holding), which increases intrathoracic & intra-abdominal pressure; avoid neck & hip flexion positions; avoid physical restraints unless absolutely necessary & ordered (fighting & restlessness increase ICP);

— administer antiemetics PRN to reduce nausea & vomiting;

— give stool softeners & make dietary adjustments to avoid constipation & giving enemas;

— give antipyretics (acetaminophen) suppositories PRN; avoid excess blankets, keep room cool (hyperpyrexia increases ICP); use hypothermia measures PRN;

— employ optimal aseptic technique & infection control measures; change insertion site dressings daily for all tubing (CVP, IV, ICP screw, ventricular catheter, etc.); use Betadine, Polysporin, or similar antibiotic ointment;

— check pt.'s eyes for corneal irritation or conjunctivitis; irrigate eyes with artificial tears, NS, or other suitable solution Q2H & place eyepads over eyes (sometimes lids have to be taped or sutured closed);

— if CSF drainage from ears or nose, cover with sterile gauze pad, but do not pack openings since this will increase pressure; do not permit pt. to blow nose; know that antibiotics are administered prophylactically to prevent meningitis;

— if steroids are used, watch for GI bleeding & other associated side effects (see NCPG #5:43, "Drugs: Corticosteroids"); administer antacids Q2H (usually by NG tube);

— if hypothermia is used, monitor & assess pt.'s condition constantly; provide good skin care & careful protection to prevent damage from circulatory stasis; know that chlorpromazine (Thorazine) PRN is often ordered to decrease shivering (avoid IM & SQ injections because of poor absorption & possible sterile abscess formation); rewarm very gradually over 24–48 hours to prevent shock caused by the body's demand for O_2 overwhelming the cold heart;

— keep close family members & friends honestly informed of pt.'s progress, prognosis, & current plan of treatment; ensure that informed consent of nearest kin has been obtained for emergency surgical intervention PRN; encourage family members & close friends to sit near pt. holding hand or stroking since there is evidence to indicate this causes a drop in ICP.

Discharge Planning and Teaching Objectives/Outcomes

1) (Patient/Family/Significant Other) Refer to NCPG #4:01, "The Patient with an Acute Head Injury," or #4:18, "The Child with an Acute Head Injury," or prepare referral forms and records for transfer of patient to convalescent hospital or rehabilitation center.

Recommended References

'Caring for the Patient With Elevated Intracranial Pressure." *Nursing 82*, January 1982:48, 49.
"Drugs: Corticosteroids." *NCP Guide #5:43*, Nurseco, Inc., 1981.
"Glasgow Coma Scale," by C. Jones. *American Journal of Nursing*, September 1979:1551–1553.
"Increased Intracranial Pressure in the Pediatric Patient: Nursing Assessment and Intervention," by C. Zeidelman. *Journal of Neurosurgical Nursing*, March 1980:7–10.
"Increased Intracranial Pressure: When Assessment Counts," by A. Ladyshewsky. *Canadian Nurse*, October 1980:34–37.
"Intracranial Pressure Monitoring Made Easy," by J. Riley. *RN*, September 1981:53–57.
Memory Bank for Hemodynamic Monitoring, by G. Ervin and S. Long. Pacific Palisades, CA: Nurseco, 1983.
"The Patient with an Acute Head Injury." *NCP Guide #4:01*, 2nd Ed., Nurseco, 1983.
"Performance Check Lists: An Effective Method of Teaching, Learning and Evaluating," by C. McCaffrey. *Nurse Educator*, January/February 1978:11–13.
"Planned Periods of Rest in the Intensive Care Unit: Nursing Care Activities and Intracranial Pressure," by M. Bruya. *Journal of Neurosurgical Nursing*, August 1981:184–193./Fl"Understanding the Signs of Intracranial Pressure—A Bedside Guide," by M. Young. *Nursing 81*, February 1981:59-62.
"Update: Head Injuries," by R. Connolly and G. Zewe. *Journal of Neurosurgical Nursing*, August 1981:195-201.
"When You're Faced With a Neuro Patient," by B. Ramirez. *RN*, January 1979:67–70.

The Patient Undergoing Intracranial Surgery: Craniotomy, Craniectomy, or Cranioplasty

Definition: "Craniotomy" is an opening in the skull to form a bone flap. "Craniectomy" is a removal of part of the skull to form a hole(s) of varying size. "Cranioplasty" is the placement of a bone graft or synthetic plate to repair a defect or opening in the skull.

LONG TERM GOAL: The patient will recover successfully from intracranial surgery and will rehabilitate as fully as possible within limitations, resuming normal or adjusted roles in family/home/society; *OR* the patient will have his vital functions maintained and be sustained with comfort and dignity until death occurs.

General Considerations:

— **Aims of surgical intervention** are to relieve intracranial pressure (ICP); to evacuate hematomas or fluid; to obtain biopsy specimens; to explore for cause of neurological dysfunction; to remove neoplasms; or to repair cerebral aneurysms, vascular anomalies, severed nerves, or fracture injuries.

— **Preoperative nursing responsibilities** include

1) reinforcing explanations and psychologic supportive measures (encouraging both patient and family to identify and air feelings) provided by the neurosurgeon; content areas should include a clear, lay description of the operation and its purpose; an honest appraisal of probable and possible anticipated results including residual neurologic deficits that may persist indefinitely; reasons for head shave and the possibilities of postoperative wigs or hairpieces;
2) obtaining a detailed assessment of baseline data for use in evaluating the patient's physiologic and mental status postoperatively; refer to NCPGs #4:01, "The Patient with an Acute Head Injury," for neurological observation and assessment, #4:11, "The Patient with Actual/Potential Increased Intracranial Pressure," for observation and assessment of IIP; and #4:41, "Assessment of Mental Status;"
3) assisting in the physical and psychologic preparation of the patient and family for diagnostic tests, which often include tomography, skull films, spinal tap, audiometry, brain scan, eletroencephalography, echoencephalography, pneumoencephalography, and/or cerebral arteriography;
4) carrying out standard preoperative activities: prep operative site—shave all or part of head as ordered; save and label hair for possible postoperative use; shampoo head gently but thoroughly with antibacterial soap recommended by your hospital; record lesions, abrasions, and infections; cover head with a clean towel or cap; refer to NCPG #2:44, "General Pre-op Nursing Care;" and

5) assisting with insertion of arterial and CVP lines for continuous monitoring; placing NG tube (see NCPG #5:46, "Nasogastric Intubation: General Principles") and long, anti-embolism stockings on patient as ordered.

— **Postoperative nursing responsibilities include**

1) carrying out standard nursing measures to support pulmonary, cardiovascular/renal, and auxiliary functions; refer to NCPGs #2:41-43, "General Post-op Care, Parts A, B, and C;" and
2) monitoring patient to ensure adequate neurologic functioning and an uncomplicated convalescence.

Specific Considerations, Potential Patient Outcomes, and Nursing Actions:

1) Neurologic Function — The patient's neurologic status will be continually monitored for changes indicative of a need for intervention; early signs of increasing intracranial pressure will be identified and reported immediately:

— refer to NCPG #4:11, "The Patient with Actual/Potential IIP," for neurologic observations & assessment;
— monitor & record vital signs Q15 minutes until stable, then QH; observe cardiac monitoring;
— monitor ICP via intraventricular catheter; record & report abnormal changes;
— have trachostomy set & mechanical ventilator readily available; check O_2 administration & maintain adequate airway; suction secretions PRN; know that cerebral hypoxia & increased CO_2 levels lead to cerebrovascular congestion & IIP, & may cause seizures;
— know that post-op positions are limited by the site of surgery & the specific restrictions imposed by the neurosurgeon; make absolutely sure that all care givers & family members clearly understand the permitted positions, head elevations, & bed adjustments;
— employ seizure precautions (padded bed rails, endotracheal tube, & padded tongue blade available, close observation, & member of family or staff in constant attendance); avoid jarring of bed or careless movement of pt.; avoid using restraints (which upset pt. & contribute to restlessness); keep room quiet & darkened;
— be alert for nocturnal seizures due to increased pCO_2 levels & falling arterial O_2 tension, which frequently occur during sleep; give anticonvulsant meds as ordered but know these may increase sleepiness & respiratory depression;
— be alert for seizures following administration of bronchial dilators & IPPB treatments; monitor closely & be prepared for cardiopulmonary arrest;
— talk to pt., re-orient him to surroundings, procedures, ongoing events; keep family informed of pt. status so they may help in calming & reassuring pt. PRN; remind them that recovery from moderate head injury & intracranial surgery is sometimes quite slow, taking weeks & months to regain functions.

2) Maintenance of Vital Functions and Prevention of Complications

The patient's life will be maintained, if possible, and further neurologic deterioration will be prevented, if possible; the patient will maintain adequate levels of fluid and electrolytes, cardiopulmonary function, elimination, and activity; the patient will be free of infection and preventable complications:

- refer to NCPG #4:01 and #4:11 for nursing actions to prevent complications;
- Keep fresh ice bags applied to head but avoid getting dressings wet;
- give analgesics (usually aspirin or acetaminophen) PRN as ordered for headache (normally present for at least 48 hours or so); know that antipyretics will also be given PRN Q4H for temp over 101°F (38.3°C);
- check dressings frequently (at least Q30 minutes); note, measure, & describe all drainage, report leakage of CSF STAT to neurosurgeon; reinforce wet dressings with dry, sterile gauze pads & expandable bandage using aseptic technique; know that, later on, when all dressings are removed, hydrogen peroxide or an antiseptic can be used to clean scalp; have available for use at that time, wigs, scarves, or muslin ski-type caps, not only for aesthetic reasons but also to conserve body heat;
- provide care for eyes to prevent corneal irritations, dryness, & periocular edema; use artificial tears, NS, ophthalmic lubrication ointment, or other appropriate medication with eye pads & small ice packs;
- monitor & record I&O carefully; administer parenteral therapy as ordered;
- keep Foley catheter unkinked & patent; provide standard indwelling catheter care; check urine specific gravity QH for 48 hours post-op or as ordered;
- keep NG tube patent to prevent vomiting (which increases ICP); observe carefully for adequate swallowing & tolerance of oral fluids when first allowed;
- give stool softeners & make dietary adjustments to avoid constipation & giving enemas (both increase ICP);
- give mouth care Q2–4H with saline or peroxide swabs (glycerine is thought to increase crusting); clean tongue & teeth; apply cream to nostrils & lips;
- use standard decubitus prevention measures; massage & protect bony prominences;
- use aseptic techniques & infection control measures; change insertion site dressings daily on all tubing (CVP, IV, ICP monitoring catheter or screw, etc.); use Betadine, Polysporin, or similar antibiotic ointment;
- position pt. strictly as ordered & change position QH gently & carefully; log roll to keep body straight & in functional alignment; avoid neck & hip flexion positions (these increase ICP);
- with surgeon's approval, perform range-of-motion exercises at least 2 x/day, but do not permit isometric exercises, pushing against footboard, or breath-holding when being moved (these efforts increase ICP);

— assist with ambulation when permitted since dizziness & disorientation are common; know that canes & walkers may be needed indefinitely throughout lengthy rehabilitation;

— keep close family members & friends honestly informed of pt.'s progress, prognosis, & plan of treatment; encourage them to assist with pt. care whenever possible & to spend as much time as possible with pt., to talk with pt., to play their favorite music or inspirational tape recordings for stimulation; remind them that comatose pts. can hear & often understand; that pts. are soothed by familiar voices & sounds;

— when pt.'s condition has sufficiently stabilized & improved enough to implement rehabilitation measures, consult with family to plan a realistic & appropriate program; help them to think through the decisions regarding practical arrangements & adjustments that must be made for each member of the family (be sure to include all siblings, nearby grandparents & step-parents as well as close friends able & willing to help); initiate suitable referrals for social services, therapy, home care, & family counseling.

Discharge Planning and Teaching Objectives/Outcomes

1) (Patient/Family/Significant Other) Has received written instructions and verbalizes understanding and acceptance of convalescent status with restrictions. Has received referral phone numbers of home health service, social service disability office, homemaker service, and other appropriate community resources. Has written appointment date and time for medical follow-up.
2) Knows medications, dosages, indications, and side effects to be reported. Has list of speech, writing, and physical exercises to be performed daily.

Recommended References

"Assessment of Mental Status." *NCP Guide #4:41*, 2nd Ed., Nurseco, 1983.
"Central Venous Pressure Line." *NCP Guide #2:40*, 2nd Ed., Nurseco, 1980.
"General Postoperative Nursing Care: Parts A, B, & C." *NCP Guides #2:41–43*, 2nd Ed., Nurseco, 1980.
"General Preoperative Nursing Care." *NCP Guides #2:44*, 2nd Ed., Nurseco, 1980.
"Intra-operative Aneurysm Clipping," by D. Morris. *Journal of Neurosurgical Nursing*, June 1982:150–153.
"Nasogastric Intubation: General Principles." *NCP Guide #5:46*, Nurseco, 1981.
"The Need For Surgical Treatment: The Patient With A Localized Mass," from "Acute Head Injury: What To Do When . . . And Why," by J. Kunkel and J. Wiley. *Nursing 79*, March 1979:29–33.
"Neurological Deficit After Carotid Endarterectomy," by P. Webb. *American Journal of Nursing*, April 1979:654–658.
"The Patient with Actual/Potential IIP." *NCP Guide #4:11*, 2nd Ed., Nurseco, 1983.
"The Patient with an Acute Head Injury." *NCP Guide #4:01*, 2nd Ed., Nurseco, 1983.
"To Sharon, With Love," by M. Cannon. *American Journal of Nursing*, April 1979:642–645.
"Treating Subarachnoid Haemorrhage Using Carotid Ligation," by D. Allan. *Nursing Times*, August 5, 1981:1383–1385.

The Patient with Leukemia

Definition: Leukemia is a neoplastic disorder of the blood-forming system resulting in an overproduction of immature, white blood cells.

LONG TERM GOAL: The patient will adhere to treatment regimen, living within restrictions, and will adjust to actual/potential losses.

General Considerations:

— **Types:** classified according to the *type or origin of white blood cell involved* and if *acute* or *chronic* (refers to maturation level of predominant cell type; acute = immature; chronic = more mature). The predominant types are:

- *lymphoblastic/lymphocytic leukemia, acute (ALL) and chronic (CLL)*; immature lymphocytes predominate (lymphatic origin); and
- *myelogenous/granulocytic/myelocytic leukemia, acute (AML) and chronic (CML)*; immature granulocytes predominate (bone-marrow origin).

— **The leukemic process:** large numbers of immature WBCs of the predominant type involved proliferate in the body, drastically reducing the normal components of the blood and causing hypertrophy of the tissue producing the cell type (e.g., splenomegaly). This results in anemia and increased susceptibility to infection and hemorrhage. Rapid destruction of cells produces an increased amount of uric acid that can result in kidney failure.

— **Occurrence:** *ALL* occurs mainly in children (for further information on this type, see NCPG #4:26, "The Child with Leukemia"); *AML* can occur in all ages, is most frequent in young adults, and is probably the most malignant of all neoplastic diseases. *CLL* and *CML* are mainly diseases of adults.

— **Signs and symptoms** usually develop over a few weeks in the acute leukemias; over many months in the chronic leukemias.

- *ALL:* fatigue, pallor, bleeding tendencies, persistent infections
- *AML:* onset of signs and symptoms may coincide with an acute URI (sore throat, fever, weakness, fatigue); bleeding tendencies
- *CLL:* uremia, weight loss, hepatomegaly and/or splenomegaly, palpable lymph nodes, lymphocytosis, anemia
- *CML:* malaise, fatigue, sweating, heat intolerance; later symptoms include abdominal discomfort, splenomegaly

— **Cause** of leukemia is unknown; some predisposing factors are exposure to radiation, chemical, and infectious agents; viruses;

genetic abnormalities; and immune incompetence.

- **Prognosis:** adult survival averages are: ALL, two to three years; AML, 10 to 12 months; CLL, five years; CML, three years. The prognosis for the lymphatic leukemias is significantly better than for the myelogenous ones.
- **Treatment** of the acute leukemias focuses on reducing and eliminating the neoplastic cells in the body. The regimen is a vigorous combination of chemotherapy, immunotherapy, and radiation, usually lasting a year or more; divided into three phases, remission induction, remission consolidation, and remission maintenance. It is usually accompanied by distressing side effects such as recurrent infections and bleeding (a result of bone marrow suppression), nausea and vomiting, and hair loss. Initial treatment begins in the hospital and lasts several weeks to months; later the patient may be discharged home on a maintenance program. Bone-marrow transplant is being used with increasing frequency.
- **Nursing responsibilities** include minimizing the many severe side effects of treatment; reducing susceptibility to infection and hemorrhage; helping patient/family/significant other (SO) adapt to loss of role of a well person and to changes in life-style; and coordinating patient care with other hospital departments.

Specific Considerations, Potential Patient Outcomes, and Nursing Actions:

1) Susceptibility to Infection — The patient will be free of hospital-based infections; the patient and family will carry out measures to prevent infections:

- know & explain that leukemic pts. have a high susceptibility to infections because their normal physiologic defenses have been drastically reduced or even eliminated (leukemic cells provide no defense against infection);
- isolate from persons with an infectious disease (some treatment regimens require strict reverse isolation); maintain a hygienic environment & carry out medical asepsis; prevent contact between pt. & staff or visitors who have URIs or other infections;
- monitor vital signs & be aware of changes that may indicate an early infection (e.g., increased TPR); avoid rectal temps since damaged mucosa is a site for bacteria;
- examine skin & mucous membranes QD for any lesions or breaks; provide mouth care several times daily; maintain good skin turgor by applying lotion to intact skin;
- teach pt. measures to ward off infections, e.g., adequate nutrition, rest & sleep, protection from physical injuries, cleanliness, avoidance of crowds & drafts.

2) Increased Risk of Hemorrhage	The patient will be monitored for early signs of hemorrhage; the patient will take precautions to reduce risk of bleeding: — know that leukemic pts. have an increased tendency to bleed due to a lowered platelet count (platelets have been crowded out by the immature WBCs); platelet transfusions may be ordered; — use small gauge needles for all injections & apply pressure dressing to puncture site after needle removal; — inspect skin & mucous membranes while giving daily care to detect signs of bleeding; instruct pt. to blow nose gently; — examine all urine & stools for gross evidence of bleeding; avoid rectal temps & medications; chart & report any changes; — use a soft toothbrush to prevent gum bleeding; give frequent oral hygiene with a nonirritating mouthwash; assess gums & oral mucosa for discomfort & bleeding; — avoid aspirin or aspirin-containing products; — know normal parameters of blood cell constituents & monitor pt.'s blood studies for changes & abnormal results; — be alert for CNS symptoms resulting from intracranial hemorrhage; — know that pt. may bruise easily; handle gently; change position carefully; refrain from pulling pt. against bed sheets; — instruct pt. about avoiding injuries; keep floor clear of objects that could cause a fall; — assess what pt. knows about transfusions (RBCs & platelets) & teach PRN (providing information can help lower anxieties).
3) Nutrition	The patient will ingest adequate food to maintain physiologic functioning and normal weight; the patient will adhere to prescribed diet: — weigh weekly & chart; — allow family members to be present at mealtimes & to help with feeding PRN; involve pt./family/SO in menu selection; — make breakfast as high in caloric intake as possible (pts. often lose their appetite as the day progresses);

- eliminate foods that cause irritation to mucous membranes; give soft foods, avoiding tough, irritating ones; avoid hot liquids;
- consult with MD & dietician regarding specific nutritional needs, e.g., increased protein, decreased calcium intake; discuss these with pt./family; assess their level of knowledge about adequate nutritional principles & teach PRN;
- provide between-meal protein supplements (eggnogs, milkshakes, etc.);
- schedule meals around chemotherapy, give oral hygiene prior to meals; control nausea with antiemetics.

4) Anxiety and Fear

The patient will verbalize decreased feelings of anxiety and fear related to the diagnosis, hospitalization, and initiation of treatment:

- assess pt.'s understanding & acceptance of illness, need for hospitalization, & planned therapy;
- assess pt.'s readiness & level of intelligence in order to plan teaching regimen;
- plan short sessions with the pt. (& family, if possible) to explain the process of leukemia, the therapeutic action & side effects of the treatment, what can be done to alleviate these;
- spend time with the pt. encouraging expression of feelings, but don't push; let pt. set own pace; accept negative feelings & know that this is part of the process of working through & dealing with the diagnosis;
- reassure pt. as to benefits of treatment (may require a great deal of support & comfort to withstand severe side effects such as nausea & vomiting, fever, etc.).

5) Psychosocial Adjustment (to Loss of Wellness and to Body Changes)

The patient will deal adaptively with changes in body image and usual role functioning; the patient/family/SO will express (and staff will accept without judgment) any and all feelings, including negative ones and those dealing with death:

- refer to NCPGs #1:27, "Impending Death;" #1:31, "Responses to Loss;" & #2:29, "Body Image Disturbance;"
- assess pt./family/SO for stage of grieving & their responses; support adaptive responses (remember that almost any response may be adaptive in the initial stage, except homicidal or suicidal behavior);
- support a realistic assessment of the situation; encourage pt. & family to plan for 1 day at a time;
- help pt. maintain a positive self-image by experimenting with wigs or hair pieces & by meeting other pts. who have successfully handled body-image changes;

— recognize the pt.'s need for unique, personal adjustments to change; support these;
— point out any signs of progress or positive change;
— arrange a staff conference to support one another; call in a mental health nurse or clinician to help staff cope with leukemic pts.

6) Drug Therapy The patient will know actions and potential side effects of drugs s/he is receiving; the patient will remain as free as possible from side effects and toxicity:
— refer to NCPG #4:44, "Drugs: Antileukemic;"
— read about specific drugs pt. is receiving in PDR or drug literature; become knowledgeable about their actions, side effects, toxic manifestations, etc.;
— report any sharp, sudden decrease in WBCs (may indicate a need to decrease the drug(s));
— provide supportive & comfort measures for pronounced side effects (minimizing these side effects requires much nursing time & skill);
— teach pt./family/SO drug actions, possible side effects, & to report any early signs.

Discharge Planning and Teaching Objectives/Outcomes

1) (Patient/Family/Significant Other) Knows to report promptly to doctor/clinic any evidence of bleeding, and if bleeding does occur, to apply pressure and go to hospital. Verbalizes a willingness to guard against injury.
2) Has a written list of medications, with times, dosage, and possible side effects. Knows toxic manifestations and methods to minimize them.
3) Can identify methods of avoiding cross-infection, can carry out reverse isolation in home; understands reasons for preventing infection, avoiding exposure to inclement weather, and for getting adequate rest. Knows to contact doctor/clinic for any signs of infection.
4) Can select a diet specific to nutritional needs. Knows to avoid foods irritating to GI tract mucosa.
5) Can verbalize some feelings about leukemia, changes in life-style, roles; is coping adaptively.
6) Has information/referral to a community support group; has an appointment for medical follow-up with doctor/clinic, and a referral for home health nursing or homemaker service PRN.

Recommended References

"The Child with Leukemia." *NCP Guide #4:26*, 2nd Ed., Nurseco, 1983.
"Dealing with Impending Death." *NCP Guide #1:27*, 2nd Ed., Nurseco, 1980.
"Drugs: Antileukemic." *NCP Guide #4:44*, 2nd Ed., Nurseco, 1983.
"Leukemia: Part I: A Hematology Review," by N. Houlihan. *Cancer Nursing*, February 1981:61-71.
Part II: "The Leukemic Process," by N. Houlihan. *Cancer Nursing*, April 1981:149-160.
Part III: "The Treatment of Leukemia," by A. Freeley and N. Houlihan. *Cancer Nursing*, June 1981:233-245.
Part IV: "The Acute and Chronic Leukemias," by A. Feeley and N. Houlihan. *Cancer Nursing*, August 1981:323-338.
Part V: "Nursing Management," by A. Feeley and N. Houlihan. *Cancer Nursing*, October 1981:397-405.
"Nutritional Problems in Radiotherapy Patients," by J. Rose. *American Journal of Nursing*, July 1978:1194-1196.
"The Patient with a Body Image Disturbance." *NCP Guide #2:29*, 2nd Ed., Nurseco, 1980.
"Responses to Loss: The Grief and Mourning Process." *NCP Guide #1:31*, 2nd Ed., Nurseco, 1980.

The Patient with Meningitis and/or Brain Abscess

Definition: *Meningitis* is an inflammation of the membranes of the brain and spinal cord. *A brain abscess or cerebral abscess* is a severe focal infection within the brain with a suppurative process. *Encephalitis* is an infection of the brain substance. *Myelitis* describes an inflammation or infection of the spinal cord. Overlap of these conditions is common and terms like meningo-encephalitis or encephalomyelitis may be used.

LONG TERM GOAL: The patient will regain optimal health with minimal neurological disability and will resume former roles in home/family/society.

General Considerations:

— **Incidence:** highest in children under two and adults over 60, although all age groups are susceptible.

— **Signs and symptoms:** high fever, severe headache, nausea, vomiting, nuchal (neck) rigidity (also shoulders and back), photophobia, confusion, irritability, ataxia, lethargy, delirium, convulsions; sometimes petechial rash (in 50% of meningococcal meningitis cases); a positive Brudzinki's sign (reactive flexion of knees and hips when patient's neck is bent forward), and a positive Kernig's sign (painful resistance during attempts to straighten patient's leg after flexing thigh toward abdomen). Specific symptoms for patient with a brain abscess include headache localized over site of abscess and tenderness over that area of the scalp. Symptoms associated with cerebral edema and increased intracranial pressure (IIP) are also commonly present.

— **Causes of meningitis** include bacterial (N. meningitidis, H. influenzae, pneumococcus, and E. coli are most common; streptococcus, staphylococcus, Tb, Klebsiella, and proteus are also seen), viral (echovirus, Coxsackie virus, communicable disease viruses are common), yeast (inhalation of Cryptococcus neoformans associated with pigeon excreta), and sometimes parasites and fungi. Onset and severity of meningitis varies from the meningococcal type (if untreated may proceed to shock, cardiopulmonary arrest, and death) to the milder, briefer illness of viral meningitis. Often there is a recent history of respiratory infection, otitis media, a chronic underlying disease, or immunosuppression.

— **Causes of brain abscess** include meningitis; septicemia; infections of mastoids, ears, sinuses, lungs, or other organs; and infections resulting from cranial puncture wounds or fractures. Organisms most commonly identified in brain abscesses are streptococcus, staphylococcus, E. coli, Klebsiella, pneumococcus, and proteus.

— **Diagnostic tests** are performed immediately upon admission and during and following the course of treatment to ascertain the cause, process, and aftermath of the infection. Tests normally include lumbar puncture (except in cases of suspected IIP), CSF culture and sensitivity, blood analysis and culture, radionuclide brain scan (for possible brain abscesses), CT scan, angiography, and electroencephalography. Cultures of other body discharges may be needed to identify the causative organism. Baseline liver and renal function studies may be done for comparison with post-antibiotic status. Serum electrolytes, urinalysis, and chest x-ray provide additional information about possible complications present upon admission or shortly thereafter.

— **Treatment and nursing responsibilities** include a careful patient assessment (a physical exam to discover diagnostic signs and a thorough history identifying recent association with other sick people, overcrowded environments, recent medications, recent illnesses or injuries); specific, closely monitored antimicrobial therapy; supportive measures to maintain vital functions, to prevent complications, and to provide comfort; infection control measures; and patient/family education to allay fears and to prepare them for continuing care at home. Sometimes brain abscesses are drained or removed surgically (refer to NCPG #4:12, "The Patient Undergoing Intracranial Surgery").

Specific Considerations, Potential Patient Outcomes, and Nursing Actions:

1) Infection Control	The patient's infection will be controlled and prevented from spreading to others in contact with patient: — place pt. in a private room; use standard isolation procedures (i.e., gowns, masks, safe disposal of secretions & needles, proper handwashing practices) for prevention of spread of airborne & direct contact organisms; — instruct family & friends re: necessity & procedures for infection control; — know that all high-risk contacts should have chemoprophylaxis for meningococcal meningitis; check with MD for orders regarding recommended drugs (Rifampin and meningococcal polysaccharide vaccine); — give antibiotics specific to causative organism identified as ordered; observe for untoward signs related to type of antibiotic administered; — monitor blood counts for depression of leukocytes or platelets; watch urine for hematuria & casts; explain to pt. & family necessity of daily lab tests; — note & report persistent or recurrent fever; consider & observe for phlebitis at IV site, pressure sore infections, cystitis, aspiration pneumonia, or other signs of nosocomial infection.
2) Maintenance of Vital Functions with Prevention of Complications	The patient will maintain adequate levels of fluids, electrolytes, and nutrition; sufficient urinary output and regular elimination; optimal cardiopulmonary and neurological status; functional musculoskeletal and integumentary system, with a minimum of preventable and controllable complications: — know that meningitis may stimulate an excessive production of antidiuretic hormone, known as Syndrome of Inappropriate Antidiuretic Hormone (SIADH); record I&O accurately; closely supervise rate of IV infusion; check specific gravity of urine each voiding; assess the serum sodium concentration daily; report signs of

hyponatremia;

- check vital signs Q4H & perform neurological observations & assessment to prevent & control IIP & increased intracerebral congestion & edema; refer to NCPG #4:11, "The Patient with Actual/Potential IIP;"
- take routine seizure precautions; have parenteral diazepam (Valium) & phenobarbital available;
- monitor pt.'s CVP; refer to NCPG #3:40, "Central Venous Pressure Line;"
- turn, cough, & deep breathe pt. QH; maintain an open airway; aspirate bronchial secretions PRN, but gently so as not to increase intrathoracic pressure or ICP; observe pt. carefully during IPPB treatments for signs of IIP;
- keep skin clean & dry, using standard decubitus-prevention measures; refer to NCPG #4:42, "Decubitus Ulcer (Pressure Sore) Care: Prevention and Treatment;"
- keep pt. in proper body alignment; prevent contractures; provide gentle, passive ROM *only* if ordered by MD (may cause IIP);
- if steroids given, refer to NCPG #5:43, "Drugs: Corticosteroids;"
- encourage full liquid diet with nutritional supplements after nausea, vomiting subside & when pt. can tolerate it; if hyperalimentation is used, refer to NCPG #3:50, "Hyperalimentation;"
- give stool softeners & check BMs daily; enemas & suppositories are permitted when dangers of IIP are past.

3) Pain and Discomfort

The patient will be relatively free of pain and discomfort caused by symptoms of the disease; the patient will express understanding and confidence in treatment and care:

- give analgesics & antipyretics PRN as ordered for fever & headache;
- give cool sponge baths for high fevers; hypothermia blanket may be ordered; apply ice bags to head & change PRN;
- keep room darkened, quiet, & free of unnecessary stimuli; limit visitors to 1 at a time; protect eyes from sudden, bright lights;
- explain all tests & treatments to pt. & family; encourage questions & help them express fears & feelings; share their concerns but be careful to avoid false reassurance; relapses & neurological deficits after discharge are common.

Discharge Planning and Teaching Objectives/Outcomes

1) (Patient/Family/Significant Other) States knowledge of possibility that some neurological disability (hearing loss, weakness of extremities, seizures, visual impairment) may linger indefinitely.
2) States s/he knows medications, dosage, indications, administration, and side effects to be reported.
3) Has appointment with doctor/clinic for follow-up medical check; knows that relapses are possible and will notify nurse or doctor immediately if symptoms or signs of illness return.
4) Has accepted referrals for home health nursing services, social service assistance, and/or transfer to convalescent hospital as needs indicate.

Recommended References

"Bacterial Meningitis—Disease of Young and Old," by T. Yoshikawa and D. Norma. *Consultant*, November 1981:219-231.
"Brain Abscess," by S. Wing. *Journal of Neurosurgical Nursing*, June 1981:123-126.
"A Case of Acute Fulminating Meningococcemia," by I. Nebens and B. Jackson. *American Journal of Nursing*, September 1982:1390-1393.
"Central Venous Pressure Line." *NCP Guide #3:40*, 2nd Ed., Nurseco, 1983.
"The CNS Catches It," by G. Hosking. *Nursing Mirror*, March 20, 1980:21-23.
'Decubitus Ulcer (Pressure Sore) Care: Prevention and Treatment." *NCP Guide #4:42*, 2nd Ed., Nurseco, 1983.
"Drugs: Corticosteroids." *NCP Guide #5:43*, Nurseco, 1981.
"Hyperalimentation." *NCP Guide #3:50*, 2nd Ed., Nurseco, 1983.
"Meningitis in the Pediatric Population," by D. Gaddy. *Nursing Clinics of North America*, March 1980:83-97.
"The Patient with Actual/Potential Intracranial Pressure." *NCP Guide #4:11*, 2nd Ed., Nurseco, 1983.
"The Patient Undergoing Intracranial Surgery." *NCP Guide #4:12*, 2nd Ed., Nurseco, 1983.
"A Patient with Meningococcal Meningitis," by A. McLennan. *Nursing Times*, January 3, 1980:29-31.
"Tap Twice for Meningitis." *Emergency Medicine*, June 15, 1981:61.
"Test Yourself—Bacterial Meningitis." *American Journal of Nursing*, July 1981:1338.

The Patient with a Retinal Detachment

Definition: A retinal detachment is a complete or partial separation of the sensory layer of the retina from the retinal epithelium.

LONG TERM GOAL: The patient will recover from a repair of a detached retina free of preventable complications; the patient will have a restored field of vision and near normal visual acuity; the patient will return to usual roles in home and community after a normal short convalescence.

General Considerations:

— **Incidence and occurrence:** rare in childhood, incidence increases with age, peaking in the 50s. Retinal detachment is more common in males, in the Jewish population, in those with myopia. Although only one eye is affected at a time, it is common to have a second retinal detachment in the other eye subsequently within the next few years.

— **Types:** rhegmatogenous (formerly called "primary"), spontaneously occurring detachments or holes usually caused by vitreous shrinkage and degenerative changes; nonrhegmatogenous (formerly called "secondary"), (1) exudative detachments when the separation is due to fluid development behind the retina from an inflammatory lesion, disease, tumor, or macula degeneration; or (2) traction detachments caused by pulling on the retina due to diabetic retinopathy, sickle-cell hemoglobinopathy, or retrolental fibroplasia. Direct trauma to the eye accounts for some cases of detached retina, but indirect injuries are now believed to only exacerbate pre-existing conditions for retinal separation.

— **Signs and symptoms:** painless onset of visual changes experienced as "flashing lights," "a shower of floating black spots, cobwebs, or particles," or a "veil" or "curtain" across part of the visual field. Loss of visual field progresses to large shadows and a decrease in visual acuity. When the separation is complete to the macula, only perception of light remains.

— **Treatment** is aimed at bringing the retinal layers into apposition at the site of the tear. On an outpatient basis this may be accomplished with laser photocoagulation or cryotherapy. More often, inpatient surgery is done with scleral buckling using silicone implants to indent eye wall and normalize intraocular eye pressure (also lowered when subretinal fluid is first removed). The operative procedure also involves producing a scar to seal the hole. This is done by causing a chorioretinitis with cryopexy or photocoagulation. **Preoperatively**, cyclopegic and mydriatic eye drops are instilled, the eyelashes are trimmed, and the face is cleansed with antiseptic. The head is positioned and draped and the patient receives a general anesthesia. **Postoperatively**, the patient has restricted eye and head movements (special positioning, eye patch, bedrest with BRP, turning only to unoperated side). S/he receives eyedrops (mydriatic, antibiotic, and corticosteroid) and, with appropriate instructions, is discharged in a few days.

— **Nursing responsibilities** include (1) complete and thorough preparation of the patient for the experience of temporary blindness. This includes indentification of familiar sounds in and just outside the patient's room; orientation to the physical layout of the room, introduction to the care givers (name and voice) who will be assigned; a reinforcement of the surgeon's explanation to the patient and family about the operation and its expected outcome; an explanation of hospital routine and care-giving procedure pre- and postoperatively; (2) administration of usual preoperative medications and special eye drops: a mydriatic to maintain pupillary dilation, a cyclopegic to temporarily paralyze muscles of accommodation, and an antibiotic to reduce pathogens in the conjunctiva; and (3) routine general preoperative measures, lab work, and examinations; refer to NCPG #2:44, "General Pre-op Care."

Specific Considerations, Potential Patient Outcomes, and Nursing Actions:

1) Eye Care — The patient will be free of postoperative complications (commonly infection); the patient will experience only minor eye discomfort:

- observe & report complaints of pain that do not respond to meds, any signs or symptoms of vision changes, or seeing light halos;
- record expected pain, swelling, & ecchymosis, but observe & report to MD purulent eye drainage or excessive swelling & discoloration;
- if ordered, apply cool, moist eye compresses for 15 minutes to reduce swelling & promote comfort;
- use aseptic technique when cleansing eye, instilling eye drops, & changing dressing; teach family member or friend how to do this when pt. goes home.

2) Comfort and Movement — The patient will be free of hypostatic pneumonia and venous stasis; the patient will comply with temporary activity restrictions and head position needs:

- position according to MD's instructions, usually with head of bed elevated & a restriction from turning to operated side;
- avoid startling pt. or bumping bed; tell pt. to avoid squeezing eyelids or moving eye under bandage; ask pt. to try, if possible, not to cough or sneeze;
- keep light in room to a minimum to reduce glare & eye squinting of unoperated eye (as well as operated eye when dressing is changed);
- observe closely for post-op nausea & promptly administer an antiemetic PRN to prevent vomiting (which would increase intraocular pressure);

- keep bedrails up as a safety measure; keep call signal within easy reach on unoperated side of bed;
- remind pt. to remain in bed, asking for assistance to the bathroom when need arises;
- support leg circulation with slow, gentle, active exercises that include ankle movement & toe wiggling at least Q4H the 1st day post-op;
- assist pt. to ambulate beginning 2nd day post-op as ordered;
- supervise deep breathing exercises with pt. holding breath on inspiration for a few seconds; this should be done at least Q4H;
- watch for signs of restlessness; ask pt. what you can do to provide comfort;
- if pt. bilaterally eye patched, refer to NCPG #1:32, "The Patient Experiencing Sensory Disturbances."

3) Intake and Output

The patient will have normal elimination restored as soon as feasible; the patient will maintain adequate hydration and nutrition:

- record I&O; monitor IV if in place;
- note frequency of urination, recording amount & specific gravity of urine;
- offer fluids each time you are in room to encourage an adequate intake;
- record gradual resumption of full diet;
- use a colon tube to relieve flatus; employ a suppository or laxative PRN to prevent constipation; avoid straining at defecation to prevent increase in intraocular pressure.

Discharge Planning and Teaching Objectives/Outcomes

1) (Patient/Family/Significant Other) Can state surgeon's instructions for eye care and has a written set of these instructions to review as needed:
   - Wash hands; clean around eye with sterile eye pad, using tepid water, wiping gently over closed eyelid from inner to outer corner; instill eye drops without touching dropper to eyelid, by pulling down lower lid, then placing one drop along inside of lower lid margin; tape eye pad in place snugly without pressure on eye.
   - Avoid showers, shampoos, contact sports, heavy lifting, or strenuous housework and yardwork for at least one to two weeks. May bathe in tub if care is taken to prevent leaning over or sudden movements. Do not bend head below waist. Bend at the knees to reach something on floor. May have hair washed in beauty salon if care is taken to avoid splashing in eye and jostling head.
   - No reading or close handwork the first week or 10 days, unless doctor permits.

2) Knows s/he can climb stairs, watch television, go for short walks, dress, and cook for self.
3) Knows to wear eye patch at night to discourage rubbing or pressure; this practice should be continued for two weeks.
4) Has a follow-up appointment with surgeon and knows to bring eye drops with him.
5) Knows to expect some eye discomfort, usually relieved with aspirin, but to immediately report sharp or persistent eye pain, sudden loss of vision, or purulent eye discharge. Knows that some floating black spots and light flashes may be experienced & persist indefinitely.

Recommended References

"Caring for the Patient with a Primary Retinal Detachment," by J. MacFayden. *American Journal of Nursing*, May 1980:920, 921.
"General Preoperative Nursing Care." *NCP Guide #2:44*, 2nd Ed., Nurseco, 1980.
"The Patient Experiencing Sensory Disturbances." *NCP Guide #1:32*, 2nd Ed., Nurseco, 1980.
"Retinal Detachment," by R. Markham. *Nursing Mirror*, February 26, 1981:xix-xviv.
"Retinal Detachment and Vitrectomy: Nursing Care," by H. Boyd-Monk. *Nursing Clinics of North America*, September 1981:433-451.

The Patient with Tuberculosis

Definition: Tuberculosis is an infectious disease caused by Mycobacterium tuberculosis. It most commonly affects the respiratory system (approximately 85% of cases) but may invade other organs of the body, such as bone, meninges, or genitourinary system.

LONG TERM GOAL: The patient will recover completely from tuberculosis, free of complications, and will resume usual roles in home/family/community.

General Considerations:

— **Incidence and occurrence:** tuberculosis (Tb) has been a major public health problem for centuries and, worldwide, is still the leading cause of death from infectious disease, affecting nearly 30,000 annually in the US alone. The disease most often occurs among adults who have a reactivation of a dormant infection.

— **Predisposing factors** that increase susceptibility include malnutrition, fatigue, mental and physical stress, and crowded living conditions.

— **High infection rates** occur among adolescent females, American Indians, Eskimos, Indochinese and Cuban refugees, and those living in urban and rural poverty areas.

— **At high risk for infection** are infants and children, the elderly, those with immunosuppressive diseases (leukemia) or drug therapy (steroids and tumor chemotherapy), and those with silicosis, diabetes, or sickle-cell anemia.

— **Transmission:** the acid-fast, causative organism is transmitted from person to person by airborne droplets from coughing or sneezing; only rarely is Tb contracted from drinking contaminated unpasteurized milk or from placental transmission to fetus.

— **Prevention:** BCG, a live, attenuated vaccine, is used extensively in developing countries where risk of Tb is high. In the US, however, it is considered useful only in unusual situations; our improved living conditions and medical treatment standards make vaccination with BCG unnecessary. The active form of the disease is prevented by treating those found to have a positive skin test. The multipuncture Tine Test is used for mass screening because it is quick and easy to use. In high risk cases, the more reliable intradermal Mantoux Test is given.

— **Classification of Tuberculosis:**

0. No tuberculosis exposure: not infected (i.e., no history of exposure and a negative tuberculin skin test)
I. Tuberculosis exposure: no evidence of infection (history of exposure and a negative skin test)
II. Tuberculosis infection: free of disease (positive skin test; no symptoms, laboratory or x-ray findings of tuberculosis)

III. Tuberculosis: infected with disease (current status is described by location or site of disease, bacteriological and chemotherapeutic status, and x-ray findings).

— **Signs and symptoms** of tuberculosis are fever, night sweats, productive cough with or without bloody sputum, wheezing, or respiratory disturbances.

— **Diagnosis** is based on a positive reaction to an intradermal tuberculin skin test, pleural biopsy, chest x-ray, and laboratory studies.

— **Treatment aims** are to cure the disease, to prevent transmission, and to prevent occurrence in the Class I patient. Most Tb patients are treated on an outpatient basis with chemotherapy, good nutrition, and a balanced rest/exercise program. Infrequently, hospitalization is desirable, ordinarily for cases complicated by other medical conditions. General hospitals, rather than sanitoria, are now used. Chemotherapy, in combined dosages of bacteriocidal agents, renders patients "nontransmitters" (i.e., with negative sputums) in less than three months; see NCPG #4:45, "Drugs: Antituberculous."

— **Nursing responsibilities** include physical/psychosocial care of a patient with an acute respiratory illness (similar to NCPG #1:17, "The Patient with Pneumonia"); patient/family education; and infection control measures. The Infection Control Committee Nurse Coordinator (or Epidemiologist) reports and coordinates patient management with the local public health department, who will assume ultimate responsibility for the patient.

Specific Considerations, Potential Patient Outcomes, and Nursing Actions:

1) Chemotherapy — The patient will be free of fever and productive cough; the patient will regain appetite and sense of well-being; the patient will have at least two negative sputum smears and become noninfectious:
- teach & supervise pt./family/significant other (SO) the important points of anti-Tb drug ingestion & recording; refer to NCPG #4:45, "Drugs: Antituberculous;"
- monitor vital signs, weight, & I&O daily; observe & record pt. response to drugs;
- know & teach that ultimate success of Tb cure depends on cooperation & faithfulness of pt. adhering to long-term self-administration of daily medications;
- establish a warm, personal, trusting, & caring relationship with pt.; do not cajole or threaten.

2) Infection Control — Room air of the hospitalized Tb patient will be free of microbial contamination; the staff, visitors, and other patients will be protected from contamination:
- report suspected & diagnosis-confirmed Tb cases to your hospital infection control committee & to your local public health dept; learn & follow their policies;
- administer pt.'s chemotherapy correctly;

— institute isolation measures from the time a presumptive diagnosis is made; maintain conscientious hand-washing & good housekeeping practices by all personnel who work around a suspected or diagnosed Tb pt.; only ordinary cleanliness is needed for eating utensils, bed linens, books, or other supplies used by pt.;
— know that any private room with proper air control (nonrecirculating air conditioning & upper room ultraviolet irradiation) may be used; pt. may also share a room with another confirmed Tb pt. on chemotherapy;
— teach pt. to cover mouth *every* time s/he laughs, coughs, or sneezes & to dispose of tissues and sputum in receptacles provided; follow standard sanitary waste-disposal methods;
— mask pt.'s nose & mouth *snugly* only and whenever s/he leaves room; use masks 1 time only;
— limit visitors to immediate family & close friends; mask visitors or nursing personnel only if adequacy of air control is questionable, if exposure must be for a prolonged period of time, or if pt. is uncooperative regarding sputum disposal; gowns & gloves are *not* necessary or desirable;
— obtain sputum specimens for C&S studies when ordered; be certain that sputum is reliable, that is, diagnostic sputum from the tracheobronchial tree obtained by a slow, forceful expiratory cough after deep breathing or use of an aerosol spray;
— determine current infectious status of pt. by reviewing sputum test results for presence of acid-fast bacilli; if there is a plateau or an increase in tubercle bacilli, report promptly to MD since drug susceptibility studies are likely to be needed.

3) Patient/Family Education

The patient/family will be able to state a basic knowledge of tuberculosis, their own current status of disease and the requirements for successful recovery; the patient/family will indicate a commitment to the value of remaining in treatment for as long as medically indicated:
— assess learner level of knowledge, readiness, & the value (appropriateness) of 1-to-1 or group teaching methods for this particular pt./family/SO; establish trust, mutual respect, & a feeling of acceptance; refer to NCPG #1:49, "Teaching Patients: General Suggestions;"
— obtain & provide appropriate leaflets from local affiliate of American Lung Assn. regarding tuberculosis, skin testing, pill taking (see Recommended References);
— discuss infectiousness, methods of control, need for protection of others, need for prolonged treatment, & prospects for complete recovery (greater than 95%);
— provide written & verbal instructions regarding chemotherapy plan & drug side effects to be reported;
— discuss value & meaning of complete recovery with successful treatment; discuss responsibility pt. feels for

self & for others; reward positive responses & behavior;
- encourage questions, airing of feelings, & discussion of possible obstacles to compliance with therapeutic regimen (e.g., fear, alcoholism, poverty conditions);
- refer to social services department for resolution of family problems, financial difficulties, disability insurance, homemaker services, and/or child-care arrangements PRN.

Discharge Planning and Teaching Objectives/Outcomes

1) (Patient/Family/Significant Other) Has received, read, and discussed American Lung Association leaflets ("Tb: Can It Happen To You?" "Pills to Prevent Tb," "The Tuberculin Test . . . How it Works . . . What it Shows," and "Positive?"). Can state in own words a basic understanding of the nature of the patient's condition and an appreciation of the necessity and commitment of self and family to long-term treatment.
2) States s/he knows to take prescribed medicine regularly and faithfully for as long as the doctor has ordered. Knows to report promptly to doctor any problems or side-effects and not to wait until next scheduled check-up appointment.
3) Has someone who will be able to provide nutritious meals and opportunities for adequate rest. Plans gradual resumption of normal activities with temporary assistance as needed.
4) Has a card with date of first follow-up visit and the names and numbers of at least two nurses (Outpatient Department or Public Health) to call for questions, in addition to physician's name and number.
5) Indicates intention of continuing medical check-ups for as long as recommended. Accepts referral of public health nurse for home visits. Demonstrates responsibility for long-term self-care and treatment.

Recommended References

Diagnostic Standards and Classification of Tuberculosis and other Mycobacterial Diseases, 14th Ed., by American Thoracic Society Medical Section of American Lung Association. Reprinted from *American Review of Respiratory Disease*, March 1981.

"Drugs: Antituberculous." *NCP Guide #4:45*, 2nd Ed., Nurseco, 1983.

Introduction to Lung Disease, 6th Ed. New York: American Lung Association, 1975:34–48.

Lung Diseases of Children, by H. Evans. New York, American Lung Association, 1979:47–56.

"The Patient with Pneumonia." *NCP Guide #1:17*, 2nd Ed., Nurseco, 1980.

"Pulmonary Tuberculosis: Test Yourself." *American Journal of Nursing*, November 1981:2039.

"Tb—Can It Happen To You?" "Pills to Prevent Tb," "The Tuberculin Test . . . How it Works . . . What it Shows," and "Positive?" (public information leaflets). New York: American Lung Association.

"Tb Treatment in Short." *Emergency Medicine*, November 30, 1980:63–64.

"Teaching Patients: General Suggestions." *NCP Guide #1:49*, 2nd Ed., Nurseco, 1980.

"Tuberculosis Today: The Development, Cure and Prevention of Tb," by R. Squires. *RN*, August 1980:42–47.

The Patient with a Vein Ligation/Stripping

Definition: Varicose veins refer to the abnormally dilated, twisted veins of the legs and thighs. Incompetent valves in the deep venous system place an extra pressure load on the superficial veins, causing their distention. Surgery involves tying off at the saphenofemoral junction, then stripping or removing the greater saphenous vein from the thigh to the ankle. Superficial venous tributaries are then either resected or cauterized. (The latter method is currently preferred to shorten hospital stay and to eliminate wound sutures and scarring.)

LONG TERM GOAL: The patient will recover from a vein ligation/stripping operation free of preventable complications; the patient will return to usual roles in home/job/community with knowledge and commitment to maintain optimum circulatory function.

General Considerations:

— **Incidence and occurrence:** an average of 10%–20% of US population is affected; incidence increases with age (40%–60% of those in their 50s have varicose veins); occurs more frequently in women.

— **Cause** is unknown; predisposing factors are hereditary predisposition, congenital weakness of veins, pregnancy, obesity, occupations that involve prolonged standing or sitting in a cramped position.

— **Signs and symptoms** include leg aches, fatigue, muscle cramps, a feeling of fullness in legs, and disfigurement of legs due to dilated, twisted, darkly-colored veins.

— **Medical treatment aims** include patient education to prevent venous stasis, to promote venous return, to prevent thrombosis, and to avoid injury to legs.

— **Surgical treatment aims** include reducing possibility of thrombophlebitis and stasis ulceration, halting progression of varicosities and tissue damage, and improving appearance of legs.

— **Nursing responsibilities preoperatively** include (1) assisting with diagnostic evaluation studies for valvular competence (Doppler Detector Pressure Test, Trendelenburg Test, venography); (2) explaining leg preparation (skin prep and surgeon marks affected veins with pen) and postoperative ambulation regimen; and (3) providing general preoperative care (refer to NCPG #2:44, "General Pre-op Nursing Care").

— **Nursing responsibilities postoperatively** include (1) performing measures to promote circulation and to prevent phlebitis; and (2) providing general postoperative care (refer to NCPGs #2:41–43, "General Post-op Nursing Care, Parts A, B, and C").

Specific Considerations, Potential Patient Outcomes, and Nursing Actions:

1) Prevention of Complications
The patient will have strong inguinal and pedal pulses, warm extremities, no edema; the patient will ambulate at least 4 x/shift when awake, placing feet flat on floor; the patient will be free of preventable complications and have pain controlled:

— keep the pt.'s legs snugly & smoothly wrapped in elastic bandages from toe to groin; remove Q8H & rewrap; observe carefully & record leg pulses, color, temperature, swelling, & the bandages for excessive bleeding;
— administer analgesics liberally PRN as ordered;
— do not permit standing still, sitting (except for meals & elimination), or leg dangling on side of bed for more than a moment; gradually lengthen walking periods each time pt. is up;
— when in bed, have pt.'s legs elevated on smooth pillows or Trendelenburg bed (no gatch or knee bend).

2) Patient Education
The patient will describe leg circulation and collateral circulation accurately; the patient will promote venous return and prevent venous stasis by cooperation with ambulation regimen and by agreeing to control weight at desired level; the patient will demonstrate proper application of elastic stockings (when ordered, as use is controversial) or bandages:

— show pt. pictures of leg circulation & how collateral circulation will develop; be certain that pt. understands the very real possibility for varicosities to recur unless certain measures are conscientiously followed;
— teach pt. to avoid girdles & garters, to refrain from crossing legs or standing for long periods, to wear support stockings or pantyhose, and to elevate legs at every convenient opportunity;
— teach pt. to avoid slip-on shoes, thongs, slippers, or sandals because they promote loss of calf-muscle pumping action needed for proper venous return;
— teach pt. to avoid prolonged pressure under knees as might occur when sitting for long periods in certain type chairs; instruct pt. re hazards of sitting for long auto/plane trips (should walk 5 minutes QH);
— explain that pt. may notice areas of numbness in the legs, but that these and the bruised, discolored, lumpy areas will gradually disappear over the next several months.

Discharge Planning and Teaching Objectives/Outcomes

1) (Patient/Family/Significant Other) Understands therapeutic regimen and indicates willingness to follow it.
2) Demonstrates ability to ambulate regularly with only moderate discomfort. Knows to rest with legs elevated above the level of the

heart at least twice daily. Is willing to lengthen walks progressively to 40 minutes daily. Knows s/he should sit no longer than 30–45 minutes at a time.

3) Agrees to wear smoothly fitting elastic bandages or stockings (if ordered) for as long as recommended, nevertheless removing them twice daily to inspect for skin breakdown or impediment to circulation.
4) Knows early signs of phlebitis (redness, warmth, tenderness) and to report them immediately to doctor/clinic.
5) Has appointment with physician for postoperative follow-up check.

Recommended References

"Breaking Down in Vein," by I. Martin. *Nursing Mirror*, July 29, 1981:34, 35.
"General Postoperative Nursing Care, Parts A, B, & C." *NCP Guides #2:41–43*, 2nd Ed., Nurseco, 1980.
"General Preoperative Nursing Care." *NCP Guide #2:44*, 2nd Ed., Nurseco, 1980.
"Simplified Surgery for Varicose Veins," by J. Hinnant and J. Stallworth. *AORN Journal*, July 1981:135–150.
"Varicose Veins," by J. Iveson-Iveson. *Nursing Mirror*, September 2, 1981:37.

The Child with an Acute Head Injury

LONG TERM GOAL: The child/youth will return to his home and family as fully recovered as possible with minimal possible residual effects of acute head injury; the family will prevent future injury to the child through implementation of safety measures (if accidental injury occurred) or through counseling (if injury was caused); *OR* the child/youth will maintain stable vital functions with/without moderate complications and neurological deficits throughout lengthy rehabilitation and convalescence; the family will learn to care for the child to maximize his return to more normal functioning; *OR* the child/youth will be sustained with compassion and dignity until life support systems have been disconnected; the family will be helped to cope with loss and grief.

General Considerations:

— **Incidence:** an estimated 200,000 children annually are admitted to the hospital for evaluation of a head injury; an equal or greater number of minor head injuries are never reported and/or cared for at home. Acute head injury is one of the leading causes of death and disability among children, an estimated 3,000 deaths yearly. Children under the age of five have a higher mortality rate than those aged five to 20 years.

— **Causes:** trauma comprises the majority of head injuries in children and youths including complications during the birth process; falls from cribs, couches, tables, etc.; child abuse ("battered-child syndrome"); vehicular accidents; and injuries resulting from toys, playground equipment, sports, and games.

— **Types** of acute head injury include *direct* blow to head (due to impact after a fall or from being hit with an object) or *indirect* by acceleration or deceleration of head due to sudden jolt (often occurs in vehicular collisions). Varieties of head injuries include skull fractures, concussions, cerebral contusions, lacerations, edema, and cerebral hemorrhage (subarachnoid bleeding; brainstem bleeding; subdural, epidural, or intracerebral hematomas).

— **Concussion** is the term used for the minor, temporary loss of brain function caused by tissue shock from a jarring of the brain; severe brain damage is not present and there is a spontaneous recovery of all neurological functions within a couple of days. Common presenting symptoms in small children include crying, vomiting, transient lethargy; in older children, behavior changes may be noted as well as complaints of headache, dizziness, and fatigue. Loss of consciousness may last from a few seconds to up to 24 hours. Post-trauma loss of awareness and amnesia (for events prior to or after injury) signify a serious concussion. There may be a postconcussion syndrome, lasting for several days or weeks, involving headaches, dizziness, anxiety, fatigue, inability to concentrate, slower thinking, and emotional disturbances.

— **Contusions** involve structural alterations of the brain, longer periods of unconsciousness (compared to concussion), and residual neurological impairment.

— **Cerebral edema** is a swelling of the brain tissue within a closed cranium (although it is somewhat expandable in young children) resulting in increased intracranial pressure (IIP), which, if not promptly reduced, leads to brain damage and death.

— **Head injuries in children** are potentially more serious because their labile responses are of shorter duration, their fluid and electrolyte balance is so easily and quickly disturbed, and their cerebral tissues are more fragile than an adult's. Since youngsters with expandable skulls may have swelling without immediately noticeable signs, severe intracranial bleeding may go undetected until the child is in shock.

— **Consequences of head injury** range from no neurological disturbance to a persistent vegetative state, or death; therefore every head injury in a child must be considered potentially serious and treated promptly.

— **Diagnostic measures** include complete neurological history and physical exam, computerized tomography (CT) scans (see Recommended References) and x-rays (skull films and cervical spine series to level of C-7 and T-1, at least; chest x-ray; IVP and other x-rays for possible internal injuries). Echoencephalography and cerebral angiography (see NCPG #5:04, "The Patient Needing Angiography") are sometimes used for evaluating possible hematoma.

— **Treatment** aims to assess accurately and to diagnose quickly the nature of the head injury and its consequences; to prevent or promptly control cerebral bleeding, edema, IIP, and brain damage; and to provide correct, expert medical and nursing measures for the maintenance of vital functions and for the promotion of brain healing. Treatment may include intracranial surgery (see NCPG #4:12, "The Patient Undergoing Intracranial Surgery"). Long-term convalescent care and complete rehabilitation is planned by specialists for those children with critical head injuries who survive. Expected residual effects of spasticity, seizures, persistent neurological deficits, and psycho/social/emotional disturbances may be encountered. The outlook for improvement over the years is better for children than for adults.

— Major immediate **nursing responsibilities** include (1) ensuring an open airway and adequate respiratory function; (2) maintaining circulating blood volume and adequate cardiac output; (3) ascertaining neurological status as soon as possible and keeping neurological assessment records; (4) obtaining as accurate and complete a history as possible of the injury, its effects, any treatment received, and any previous relevant history (diseases, medications, allergies, etc.); (5) providing explanations and realistic reassurance to patient and family; and (6) preparing child (and family) for surgery, if indicated.

Specific Considerations, Potential Patient Outcomes, and Nursing Actions:

1) Neurological Observation and Assessment

The child's neurological status will be continually monitored for changes indicating a need for intervention; early signs of IIP will be identified and reported immediately:

— see this section in NCPG #4:11, "The Patient with Actual/Potential Increased Intracranial Pressure;"

— know the different levels of consciousness (LOC) & describe behavior clearly, carefully, & comprehensively, unless your hospital uses an exceptionally reliable, standardized, neurological observation record; obtain frequent (Q15 minutes) & continuing checks of LOC;

— check reflexes & note presence or absence (gag, swallow, elbow, knees, Babinski);

— check ability to speak without hoarseness or dysphasia;

— note & report bruising behind ear ("Battle's sign"), periorbital ecchymosis ("raccoon eyes"), otorrhea, or rhinorrhea (either bleeding or CSF);

— accompany pt. for CT scan in order to provide constant, consistent nursing care & monitoring, especially if pt. is a child in critical condition; explain to child (if possible) & parents what this painless, though frightening procedure entails; give necessary prescribed presedation & remain with child to note & record response;

— do not elevate pt.'s head or flex neck until spinal injury has been ruled out (cervical collar may be temporarily applied until cervical spine films are taken & diagnosis is clear); examine pt. for scalp wounds, skull lumps, or tenderness; look for CSF leakage from nose & ears; smell for alcohol on the youth's breath (this may confuse neurological assessment but not all symptoms may be alcohol related); check for symmetry & strength of reflexes; review & assess function of cranial nerves;

— ask pt., family member, witness to injury about (a) cause of injury (a missile? object striking the head? fall? auto or vehicular collision? sudden jolt?); (b) site of injury, direction and force of blow, secondary injury resulting from fall after blow; (c) any loss of consciousness? for what length of time? how aroused? any seizures before or after fall or head injury? if so, obtain as complete a description as possible; length of time since injury; behavior since injury (level of alertness or responsiveness); (d) other signs and symptoms such as bleeding from ears, nose, eyes, mouth, or elsewhere; clear fluid leakage from nose, ears, head; paralysis, loss of feeling, limpness or weakness of extremities; loss of bladder or bowel control; signs of infection; signs of fluid imbalance; vomiting; headache; amnesia, aphasia, or dysphasia; (e) treatment, drugs, alcohol taken before injury or exact treatment or medications administered before arrival at hospital after injury; history of frequent accidents, falls, head injuries, seizures, or illnesses;

— be aware of effect of medications, physical movements, or conditions which may affect ICP, mask signs or potentiate them, or make interpretation and accurate assessment more difficult;
— observe, record, & report (during succeeding days of hospitalization) aftereffects of head injury such as headache, nausea, vomiting, dizziness, emotional irritability; record type of amnesia (retrograde—events prior to injury; antegrade—events during a following injury); note presence & type of aphasia or dysphasia.

2) Maintenance of Vital Functions and Prevention of Complications

The child/youth's life will be maintained, if possible, and further neurological deterioration will be prevented; the patient will maintain adequate fluid & electrolyte levels, cardiopulmonary function, and elimination; the patient will be free of infection and preventable complications resulting from immobility and therapeutic regimen:

— see this section in NCPG #4:11, "The Patient with Actual/Potential Increased Intracranial Pressure;"
— check vital signs Q15 minutes; check for signs of bleeding & blood loss; establish IV lines for parenteral administration of glucose, blood, Ringers Lactate, volume expanders, etc.; place child on cardiac monitor; maintain arterial lines for blood gas determinations & monitoring; obtain specimens for necessary lab work (CBC, Hct., Hbg., and T&C, etc.); document I&O, vital signs, observations, & assessments;
— elevate head of bed 15°-30° to promote cerebral venous drainage by gravity;
— insert an NG tube as appropriate; if NG tube in place, keep patent; check for GI bleeding & know that ulceration is possible from stress or from glucocorticosteroids; give antacids Q2H & cimetidine as prescribed;
— know that, except for cases of hypovolemic shock, fluid intake will be restricted (sometimes to 600–1000 ml/24 hours); use microdrip IV tubing sets & monitor rate of parenteral therapy closely;
— monitor I&O carefully; record urine output & specific gravity QH; provide Foley catheter care to assure patency & prevent infections;
— pad side rails & take seizure precautions especially if child has a seizure history, a skull fracture, a suspected hematoma, or a GCS Index score of 8 or less; have parenteral forms of diphenylhydantoin (Dilantin) & diazepam (Valium) (drug choice for status epilepticus) readily available; know that the therapeutic blood level loading dose of 10 mg/Kg will last about 24 hours;
— know that the side-lying position is usually preferred for the comatose pt. to prevent aspiration & airway occlusion, but location & extent of injuries may alter this; maintain functional body alignment; avoid neck flexion positions (increases ICP); avoid hip flexion (increases intra-abdominal pressure leading to IIP); turn pt. slowly & gently, "log rolling" to keep body straight; have pt. exhale while turning to prevent Valsalva maneuver (breath holding that increases intrathoracic & intra-abdominal pressure);

- assist lab & x-ray personnel with necessary tests so child is not moved or disturbed unnecessarily or harmfully;
- protect child from injuries due to restless movements, disorientation, & seizures, but avoid physical restraints unless absolutely necessary & ordered (fighting & restlessness increase ICP); assess, report, & attempt to correct causes of restlessness (pain, a distended bladder due to a kinked or clamped catheter, tight casts or bandages, respiratory distress, bleeding, increasing ICP); if child is regaining consciousness, s/he may need a member of the family or close friend to be there; there is evidence to indicate that if they hold pt.'s hand, stroke or talk to pt., this causes a drop in ICP & pt. will be calmer; avoid unnecessary sedation that may cause respiratory depression & mask neurological symptoms;
- prevent contractures with standard measures (i.e., bed board, foot board, trochanter rolls, & devices to prevent hand deformities); give passive range-of-motion exercises (isometric exercises will increase ICP); understand & cooperate with physical therapy aims & program;
- bathe & inspect skin QD for hydration & turgor, rashes, abrasions, contusions, signs of pressure sores, infection or phlebitis at puncture sites; give soothing sensory stimulation by stroking & touching while talking to pt.;
- use standard decubitus-prevention measures (i.e., an alternating pressure pad or flotation mattress); massage & protection for heels, elbows, bony prominences, etc.;
- give mouth care Q2–4H with saline or peroxide swabs (glycerine may increase crusting); clean tongue & teeth; apply cream to nostrils & lips;
- employ optimal aseptic technique & infection control measures; change insertion site dressings QD for all tubing (CVP, IV, ICP screw, ventricular catheter, etc.); use Betadine, Polysporin, or similar antibiotic ointment;
- check pt.'s eyes for corneal irritation or conjunctivitis; irrigate eyes with artificial tears, NS, or other suitable solution, Q2H & place eyepads over eyes (sometimes lids have to be taped or sutured closed);
- keep close family members & friends informed honestly of child's progress, prognosis, & current plan of treatment; encourage them to assist with pt. care whenever possible & to spend as much time as possible with pt., to talk with child, to play their favorite music or inspirational tape recordings for stimulation; remind them that pt. can often hear & understand, that pts. are soothed by familiar voices & sounds;
- encourage pt.'s family & friends to express their fears, feelings of helplessness, guilt, anger, & despair outside the pt.'s hearing range; arrange for spiritual & emotional counseling PRN;

— support *realistic* hopes (1 study showed only 6% of patients with coma lasting longer than 2 months made any significant recovery, but there are surprising exceptions); prepare them for the prolonged care usually associated with serious head-injured pts., i.e., long-term recovery & rehabilitation; help them to think through the decisions regarding practical arrangements & adjustments that must be made for each member of the child's nuclear family (consider all siblings, nearby grandparents, & step-parents as well as close friends).

3) Patient/Family Education — The family/significant other (SO) will know observations of child to make at home; knows signs of untoward developments:

— instruct family/SO to return to hospital if:
- unable to awaken child or if child is disoriented (awaken child Q1–2H for 24 hours and ask child to give own name, where s/he is, and what happened)
- *severe* headache (give only aspirin or acetaminophen for headaches, nothing stronger; do not give sedatives, tranquilizers antihistamines, or other medications;)
- *persistent* vomiting (mild nausea and vomiting are common; give clear liquids and soups as tolerated for 1st 24 hours after head injury);
- unequal pupils or vacant, staring look in pt.'s eyes;
- weakness, limpness, or loss of feeling in arms or legs;
- any kind of seizure or stiffness in body;
- any drainage from nose or ears.

Discharge Planning and Teaching Objectives/Outcomes

1) (Child/Parents/Significant Other) Can state the normal aftereffects of an acute, *minor* head injury (headache; dizziness; *some* drowsiness and fatigue; emotional irritability and periodic euphoria or depression; difficulty speaking, remembering, computing sums, writing paragraphs) and know that these may last from a few days to a month or longer. Knows that impaired memory and delayed reaction time also may follow even a minor head injury and patient should return to former activities gradually and part-time.
2) Knows that following a *moderate* head injury, in addition to above symptoms, patient may also have episodes of hallucinations, delusions, personality alterations, cognitive disorders, sleep disturbances, and psychosocial disturbances for many months to years (over the years, most of these sequelae eventually disappear).
3) Knows (has been told) if there is a risk of seizures, so that activities of daily living can be adjusted accordingly, if desired.

4) (If child/youth is to be sent home instead of to a convalescent hospital or rehabilitation center) has reviewed a written plan for activities permitted, for exercise, diet, medication, and rehabilitation. Family is well prepared to provide appropriate care for physical and emotional needs of convalescing patient.
5) Can identify the signs of *increasing* difficulty (irrational behavior changed from pre-injury behavior, restlessness, combativeness, amnesia, disorientation, *increasing* limb weakness and difficulty walking or speaking, *increasing* drowsiness and unresponsiveness to verbal commands). Knows to seek immediate medical care without further delay.
6) Has medical appointment for follow-up medical and psychological rehabilitation and care.
7) If needed, has received social service referral for assistance with arrangements for vocational and educational assistance, community health nursing services, physical/speech/occupational therapy, and psychological counseling.

Recommended References

"Acute Head Injury: What To Do When . . . And Why," by J. Kunkel and J. Wiley. *Nursing 79*, March 1979:23–33.
"Bringing the Unconscious Patient Back Safely—Nursing Makes the Critical Difference," by N. Mauss-Clum. *Nursing 82*. August 1982:34–42.
"The Child: Battered-Child Syndrome." *NCP Guide #4:20*, 2nd Ed., Nurseco, 1983.
"Computed Tomographic Scanning of the Brain," NIH Consensus Development Conference Summary. Bethesda, MD: National Institute of Neurological and Communicative Disorders and Stroke, November, 1981.
"Concussion," by C. Fritz. *Nursing 81*, September 1981:84.
"Drugs: Corticosteroids." *NCP Guide #5:43*, Nurseco, 1981.
"Glasgow Coma Scale," by Cathy Jones. *American Journal of Nursing*, September 1979:1551–1553.
"Head Injuries—Part 1: Advances in Care During Past Decade," "Part 2: Advances in Diagnostic Equipment," by J. Young. *Nursing Times*, April 30, 1981:766-769; May 7, 1981:819-821.
"Head Trauma." *Emergency Medicine*, November 15,1980:103–105.
"Head Trauma In Children," by C. Walleck. *Nursing Clinics of North America*, March 1980:115–130.
"Life-Threatening Head and Spinal Injuries," by P. Perdue. *RN*, June 1981:36–41.
"Nursing Management of the Head Injured Patient," by J. Kunkel. *Critical Care Update*, March 1981:22–24.
"Of Course You Can Manage Head Trauma Patients," by K. Mastrian. *RN*, August 1981:44–51.
"Outcome Following Closed Head Injury," by C. Jones. *The Journal of Neurosurgical Nursing*, August 1981:178–183.
"The Patient with Actual/Potential Increased Intracranial Pressure." *NCP Guide #4:11*, 2nd Ed., Nurseco, 1983.
"The Patient Undergoing Intracranial Surgery." *NCP Guide #4:12*, 2nd Ed., Nurseco, 1983.
"Preparing Children and Parents for Cerebral Computerized Tomography," by G. Mill. *MCN: American Journal of Maternal-Child Nursing*, November/December 1980:403–407.
"Traumatic Head Injury: Restlessness and Agitation as Prognosticators of Physical and Psychological Improvement in Patients," by R. Reyes et al. *Archives of Physical Medicine and Rehabilitation*, January 1981:20–23.
"Update: Head Injuries," by R. Connolly and G. Zewe. *Journal of Neurosurgical Nursing*, August 1981:195–201.
"What To Say . . . And Do . . . When Your Patient Asks About CT Scans," by C. Haughey. *Nursing 81*, December 1981:72–77.

The Child with an Acute Respiratory Infection

Definition: *Croup* is an inflammation of the larynx and trachea, also known as laryngotracheobronchitis.
Bronchiolitis is an inflammation and obstruction of the bronchioles.
Epiglottitis is an infection of the epiglottis, aryepiglottic folds, and supraglottic area, quickly leading to airway obstruction.
Tracheitis is a swollen, infected trachea.
Influenza is a disease of the respiratory tract.
Pneumonia is an inflammation of the lungs.
Bronchopneumonia is an inflammation of the terminal bronchioles and alveoli of lungs.

LONG TERM GOAL: The child will recover optimum health free of complications and will resume normal growth and development.

General Considerations:

Type	Incidence and Occurrence	Causes	Signs and Symptoms
Croup	Occurs mainly during winter months; is one of the most common respiratory diseases in infants and young children aged three months to three years; affects boys more than girls.	Various types of viruses (often parainfluenze I, II, III) in 2/3 of cases.	Hoarse voice; deep, rasping, harsh cough; dysphagia (difficulty swallowing); sore throat; tachypnea (rapid breathing); restlessness; anxiety; inspiratory stridor (harsh airflow sound); retraction (breast bone and muscles of neck pulled in); low fever; possibly vomiting.
Bronchiolitis	Accounts for nearly half the hospitalizations for respiratory diseases in the baby under two years; average case age is five to six months.	Nearly always a virus, often the respiratory syncytial agent (RSV).	Hacky cough, nasal discharge; low grade fever, rapid respirations (above 60/minute), prolonged wheezing, anorexia.

Type	Incidence and Occurrence	Causes	Signs and Symptoms
Epiglottitis	More common in children aged two to seven years; according to some studies, is more prevalent in boys.	H. influenzae type B bacterium.	Cherry-red, inflamed sore throat to point of drooling; high fever (38.5°C/101.3°F); difficulty breathing and swallowing; increased pulse rate; cyanosis; restlessness and apprehension due to hypoxia.
Bacterial Tracheitis	Peaks in the winter months; occurs primarily in children under three years.	Staph aureus, Group A strep, and H. influenzae most common.	URI, high fever, inspiratory stridor, croupy cough.
Influenza	More common in school-age children because of epidemic nature of disease; outbreaks every one to two years.	Antigenic shifting types of viruses.	High fever (38.3°-41°C/101°-106°F), chills, headache, muscle and joint pain, malaise, nasal obstruction. cough, photophobia.
Pneumonia	Common in all age groups of children; especially seen as a complication to childhood diseases; accounts for about 5% of acute illnesses in children under 17.	Bacteria (streptococcus, staphylococcus, pneumococcus, pseudomonas, Klebsiella, other); viruses (parainfluenza, adenoviruses, RSV, rubeola, varicella, other); foreign materials (kerosene, food, dust, other small objects, lipids, chemicals); fungi, rickettsia, protozoan are occasional causes.	High fever (39.4°-40°C/103°-104°F), rapid respiration (50-80/minute), rapid heartbeat (above 100/minute) chills, dry painful cough, labored breathing, anorexia, malaise, abdominal distention, flared nostrils, chest wall retraction, often vomiting in the under-two year old or convulsions in the infant.

— **Treatment aims** are to relieve respiratory distress and to prevent complications (respiratory and cardiac arrest, atelectasis, bronchiectasis, septicemia, other) by symptomatic and supportive measures such as humidified oxygen, tracheal suctioning,

IPPB, parenteral therapy hydration, steroids. When possible, treatment aims to identify and remove causative organism. Since most respiratory infections in children are caused by viruses, antibiotics are only given when bacterial causes are known or when there is no improvement with treatment after the first few days.

— **Hospitalization is recommended** for all but the mildest cases of respiratory infection in young children because viral respiratory infections are the second leading cause of death in infants and young children. Because of the size and stage of development of respiratory tract anatomical structures, children are especially vulnerable to airway obstruction and permanent airway damage. In addition, their needs for oxygen are greater so they are at greater risk for respiratory and cardiac arrest. Whereas croup and influenza have usually run their course in less than a week, recovery from pneumonia may take at least two to four weeks or longer. In the first 24 to 48 hours, bronchiolitis, epiglottitis, and tracheitis may become medical emergencies unless quickly, skillfully, and correctly treated with intubation (nasotracheal, tracheostomy), repeated suctioning, ventilation assistance, oxygen, antibiotics, steroids, just enough sedation and restraints to prevent accidental extubation, and maintenance of hydration. Barring complications, the hospital stay ranges from seven to 14 days.

— **Nursing responsibilities** include immediately assessing respiratory and cardiac status, then other patient care needs and problems; maintaining adequate hydration; assisting with provision of supportive treatment measures; continuing observation and intervention to prevent or control complications; and alleviating anxiety in child and family.

Specific Considerations, Potential Patient Outcomes, and Nursing Actions:

1) Respiratory Function

The child will resume normal breathing pattern, maintain a patent airway, liquefy and raise secretions, and experience relief of cyanosis and apprehension related to respiratory distress:

— establish & maintain patent airway; have Ambu bag, laryngoscope, tracheostomy supplies, & emergency stimulants readily accessible; arrange for a supply of sterile endotracheal tubes (need to have those that are 1 size smaller than child's little finger to reduce risk of complications like subglottic stenosis);

— have racemic ephedrine & IPPB equipment on hand for relief of airway obstruction in croup cases; be prepared to administer treatments Q2H PRN to relieve symptoms; know that dexamethasone (steroid) may be given to potentiate effect of racemic ephedrine;

— monitor vital signs closely & frequently; observe pattern, rate, & characteristics of respirations, pulse, heartbeat; note & record clinical features of child's condition (i.e., wheezing, nasal flaring, hoarseness, drooling, cough characteristics, location & type of pain, etc.);

— be especially vigilant & report, STAT, signs of increasing airway obstruction (tachycardia, tachypnea, sitting

up or head thrust forward for mouth breathing, retraction or stridor at rest, pallor, listlessness, circumorbital or circumoral cyanosis, anxiety, restlessness (sign of hypoxia), & diminution of breath sounds);
— adjust child's position according to age & head control (use infant seat or elevate head of bed); cover to prevent chilling, but keep clothing light & loose;
— administer O_2 at prescribed concentration via face mask, tent, or assisted ventilation; observe & record child's response;
— monitor progress via assessment of blood gases analysis (CO_2 & O_2 levels);
— suction secretions PRN using aseptic technique; help older child raise secretions, coughing them into tissues, rather than swallowing mucus; splint chest to assist child in coughing productively; teach & help with postural drainage when child is able; chart frequency, amount & appearance of expectorated sputum; save specimen for analysis & culture; *NOTE: do not attempt a throat culture if diagnosis of epiglottitis is suspected, since a sudden airway closure may be precipitated*;
— if intubated, keep child sedated (carefully, so as not to further depress respiration) & properly restrained to forestall accidental extubation; if tracheostomy done, refer to NCPG #2:25, "The Patient with a Tracheostomy."

2) Infection Control

The child will respond to antibiotics as expected in bacterial infections; the child will respond to measures for control of viral infections; the child will not acquire additional, complicating infections from lowered resistance; there will be reduced incidence of nosocomial (hospital-acquired) respiratory infections for visitors and staff:
— use isolation precautions & private room until child has been afebrile for at least 72 hours;
— instruct staff & visitors to wash hands before & after handling child or entering pt.'s room;
— do not permit nursing staff or visitors with child if they are pregnant, recovering from illness or surgery, or over age 60 until all signs of acute infection have subsided;
— follow your hospital's procedure for care of respiratory therapy equipment (e.g., use of sterile liquids, aseptic suctioning technique, changing all tubing every 8–24 hours, disinfecting or sterilizing all equipment used);
— if tracheostomy, check skin & tissue around site for irritation & crust formation; cleanse with hydrogen peroxide & normal saline, blot dry;
— give antibiotics, steroids, & other medications correctly & on time to maintain therapeutic blood levels; note & chart child's response to all medications;

— prevent phlebitis & IV cutdown infections with correct aseptic IV equipment techniques;
— observe & report signs of otitis media, septicemia, atelectasis, or pneumonia (common complications of respiratory infection in children);
— change child's position regularly, taking care to keep skin clean, dry, & free of pressure & irritation.

3) Fluids and Electrolytes — The child will be adequately hydrated and have nutrition maintained; the child will have temperature return to normal; the child will have intake and output and fluids and electrolytes in therapeutic balance:
— record I&O carefully & accurately; weigh daily;
— monitor parenteral therapy for safe, accurate administration;
— record urine amount, appearance, & specific gravity with every voiding; report values of greater than 1.015 (underhydration, thickened secretions) or less than 1.008 (may indicate overhydration & increased risk of pulmonary edema);
— utilize appropriate cooling measures for temp over 39.5°C/103°F; take care to avoid chilling;
— give antipyretics as ordered; *NOTE: salicylates are usually avoided in influenza cases to reduce risk of acquiring Reye's Syndrome in susceptible children*;
— as soon as able, encourage child to take room temperature (not cold) liquids orally; gradually introduce soft food as condition improves.

4) Psychosocial Adjustment to Hospitalization — The child will have confidence and trust in the medical and nursing staff, accepting care and treatment with minimal stress; the child will adapt effectively to the stress of illness, hospitalization, and treatment via play therapy and the supportive presence of parent, relative or friend; the child and parent/significant other (SO) will cope with anxiety effectively and productively as evidenced by cooperation and participation in therapeutic regimen:
— review NCPG #3:30, "The Child with Separation Anxiety;"
— whenever possible, organize nursing measures & treatments to provide a maximum of rest for both child & parent (fatigue lowers stress management skills);
— since crying increases the child's need for O_2, encourage the parent/SO to remain with child as much as possible; help them to arrange time off for themselves while another, close to the child, temporarily relieves them;

- support & reassure parent/SO so they can effectively comfort child in a more relaxed manner; involve them in the child's care & whenever possible have the child also participate; provide simple explanations & demonstrations, patiently repeating PRN;
- encourage both parents & child to express feelings & fears; take time to listen;
- utilize play therapy to facilitate child's adjustment to hospitalization & treatment; read & sing to the child, use puppets, provide television cartoons or other shows producing laughter; refer to NCPG #3:30, "Play Therapy: General Suggestions."

Discharge Planning and Teaching Objectives/Outcomes

1) (Patient/Family/Significant Other) States s/he knows the importance of having good nutritious meals, several rest periods daily, gradual resumption of play and sports when energy returns.
2) Understands the importance of avoiding overexertion, chilling, other persons with an infection (lowered resistance may linger several weeks).
3) Knows what medications to take, possible side effects, amounts, and indication for administration.
4) Will practice blowing balloons and breathing exercises to strengthen lung expansion. Can demonstrate effective postural drainage and agrees to do it faithfully two or three times daily until chest is clear and coughing ceases.
5) States s/he realizes importance of keeping follow-up doctor's appointment, even if child feels much better and another trip to the doctor is considered inconvenient. (Airway damage is common and child may need to practice special health measures to avoid recurrences.)

Recommended References

"Acute Epiglottitis," by E. Fried. *Issues In Comprehensive Pediatric Nursing*, September-December 1980:29–35.
"The Child with Separation Anxiety." *NCP Guide #3:20*, 2nd Ed., Nurseco, 1983.
"The Crises of Bronchiolitis" and "Croup and Epiglottitis," by R. Simkins and "Pneumonia," by M. Pinney. *American Journal of Nursing*, March, 1981:514–520.
"Croup, Epiglottitis and Now Tracheitis." *Emergency Medicine* November 15, 1979:87–88.
"Humanistic Nursing Care for Critically Ill Children," by K. Stevens. *Nursing Clinics of North America*, December 1981:611–622
Lung Diseases In Children by H. Evans. New York: American Lung Association, 1979:27–47.
"Nursing Aspects of Pediatric Intensive Care in a General Hospital," by M. Soupios et al. *Pediatric Clinics of North America*, August 1980:621–632.
"The Patient with a Tracheostomy." *NCP Guide #2:25*, 2nd Ed., Nurseco, 1980.
"Pitfalls in Pediatric Pulmonology," by L. Taussig. *Emergency Medicine*, September 15, 1980:25–46.
"Play Therapy: General Suggestions." *NCP Guide #3:30*, 2nd Ed., Nurseco, 1983.
"Short-term Intubation in Children with Acute Epiglottitis," by R. Schultz and W. Morrison. *Southern Medical Journal*, February 1982:158–160.

The Child: Battered-Child Syndrome

Definition: "Battered-Child Syndrome" is the term used by hospitals to identify the victim of child abuse. Child abuse is the nonaccidental injury or neglect inflicted upon children by their care takers. It includes physical and emotional neglect, physical battering, psychologic attack, and sexual molestation.

LONG TERM GOAL: The child will experience healing, protection, and relief from pain, injury, fear, and neglect. The parents (or care takers) will obtain support in adopting methods that limit the potential for abusing their child. The parents will implement new coping mechanisms, will seek appropriate help, and will not abuse the child.

General Considerations:

— **Incidence and occurrence:** maltreatment and neglect of children is a widespread, universal social problem, occurring in both urban and rural populations, in all races, and at all socioeconomic levels. A conservatively estimated one million American children suffer from abuse and neglect. Perhaps twice this number go undetected, unreported, uncorrected. Sexual abuse accounts for at least 20% of the reported cases, but this type of abuse is commonly not reported. There is a one in four chance that a child will be a victim of child molestation, incest, or rape before the age of 18. (Refer to NCPG #4:27 "The Child Victim of Rape/Sexual Assault").

— **Common manifestations:** neglected children may be underweight or overweight (from improper nutrition), wear clothing inappropriate for weather, have infections that are not being treated, and have poor dental hygiene. Victims of battering or physical abuse may exhibit bruises, abrasions, contusions, lacerations, or welts in various stages of healing over arms, legs, or buttocks; lumps on scalp are common as are retinal hemorrhages (from shaking child); burns (from cigars or cigarettes) may be seen on soles of feet, palms of hands, buttocks, or genitalia; immersion, scalding burns of hands, feet, and buttocks may be noted; human bite marks, dental injuries, or cuts around mouth or eyes, and bald patches on scalp (where hair has been pulled out) may be seen; multiple fractures are suspicious, especially in children under two. Behaviorally, they may stare, appear unresponsive, ignore friendly overtures, perform self-stimulation activities, seek attention with asocial or delinquent acts, or miss school frequently or fall asleep in class (from assuming sibling-care responsibilities at home). Other behavioral indicators include shyness, even fearfulness at approach or touch of an adult; passivity while being examined; apprehension when hearing other children cry; verbal expectations of punishment for minor, childish accidents (such as spilling milk or wetting bed); and attention-seeking behaviors. The presence of one indicator on emergency room admission need not be necessarily viewed with alarm, but repeated "accidents" or multiple signs are a cause for suspicion and precautionary reporting.

- **Causes:** child abuse is a multidimensional, adult illness of epidemic proportions with psychopathological, behavioral, environmental, social, and cultural factors. Approximately 90% of abusers have a history of having being abused. Triggering behaviors include drug and alcohol intoxication, quarreling between adults/care takers, uncontrolled sibling rivalry, perceptions that the victim's behavior is abnormal or atypical, stressful life circumstances (divorce, unemployment, single parenting, financial worries), and other crises. Typically the abusing adult is dependent, immature, unable to handle responsibility, and a social isolate. The person often has a low self-esteem, a low tolerance for stress, and an impulsive overreaction to frustration and tension. Frequently the person has an unrealistic expectation and misconception about normal child behavior and developmental stages. S/he believes in the value of physical punishment, sees in the child's behavior a reflection of own self-worth, and looks to the child to gratify own wishes and needs. This leaves the child confused about own role and relationships, emotionally starved, and with feelings of low self-worth, hopelessness, and sadness.
- **Legal requirements for reporting child abuse and neglect:** all 50 states now have statutes requiring public officials and professional persons (including teachers, school administrators, and nurses) who work with children to notify appropriate authorities of suspected instances of physical, emotional, or sexual child abuse and/or neglect.
- **Nursing responsibilities** include:

1) becoming informed by reading recommended references, attending seminars on the subject, or writing for further information to:

National Committee for Prevention of Child Abuse
111 East Wacker Drive, Suite 510
Chicago, IL 60601

The Child Abuse League of America
67 Irving Place
New York, NY 10003

The Children's Division of the American Humane Association
P.O. Box 1226
Denver, CO 80201

National Center for the Prevention and Treatment of Child Abuse and Neglect
Dept. of Pediatrics, U of Colorado Medical Center
1205 Oneida Street, Denver, CO 80220

2) becoming concerned and involved over this growing problem: learn what local services exist; compile a resource file for use by other professionals as well as yourself; consider joining or forming a group of:
   - *VICA* (Volunteers in Child Abuse): a project involving trained volunteers for parents who need support, friendship, and role models to help their parenting skills
   - *For Kid's Sake*: an organization that helps detect and prevent child abuse

- *CALL* (Child Abuse Listening Line) or *Parents Anonymous* (PA) *Hot Line*: be a telephone volunteer
- *"P.A. Buddies"*: work with troubled parents on a one-to-one basis
- *"P.A. Sponsors"*: gives low key guidance and support to PA groups

3) reporting cases of suspected child abuse: know whether your state has permissive or mandatory legislation on reporting suspected cases; failure to report may be a crime subject to penalties and fines; persons who report in good faith are granted immunity from criminal and civil court action, even if the report proves erroneous. Carefully document all physical evidence of injury or neglect without making any judgment statements about parents or care takers; "copping out" behind a "failure to thrive" diagnosis or "accidental injury" report hurts and endangers the child as well as neglects the parent/care taker who desperately needs help; early recognition and reporting of suspected child abuse is the key to prevention of further, possibly fatal recurrences; consider the report as a first step to the helping process; and
4) working to develop within your health agency a concerted effort with policy guidelines on child abuse prevention and treatment, which will plug into your community services, avoiding duplication and wasted resources.

Specific Considerations, Potential Patient Outcomes, and Nursing Actions:

1) Observation and Assessment

The child will be accurately diagnosed:
- — note & chart unusual findings upon admission (scars, bruises, unexplained marks);
- — observe & describe suspicious behavioral characteristics (passive response to pain, fearful & withdrawn, flinching & ducking when anyone reaches out to touch, violent aggressiveness to dolls & play objects);
- — observe, assess, & record social environment of family (parents' potential for abuse & child's risk: see Recommended References for screening suggestions).

2) Protection from Injury

The child will have maximum healing, recovery, and protection from further injury:
- — monitor visitors discreetly; friendly visits with care takers can provide acceptance & diffuse hostility;
- — refer to nursing care planning guide for specific type of injury (head injury, fracture, burn, etc.);
- — make referral to hospital social service department or your local Department of Social Service, community mental health center, or child abuse prevention center;
- — know that for the child's safety & protection, s/he may be placed in temporary custody of courts, but this may increase the child's feeling of loss of parental love; know that often the child will reject your "rescue" & cling to parent; be careful not to overidentify with the child & lose your objectivity; focus upon the needs of the whole family for help; remember the best help for the child is to help the parent/care taker.

3) Psychosocial Adjustment to Trauma

The child will experience relief from pain, fear, and emotional side effects of trauma; the child will be helped to regain feelings of dignity, self-worth, and trust:

— encourage child to talk about how s/he feels; be a warm, quiet listener, avoiding judgmental comment;
— provide drawing materials (children often depict their feelings in this way); gently ask about meanings of drawings; do not probe; provide other play materials & objects for expressing feelings (puppets, doll houses, etc.); refer to NCPG #3:30, "Play Therapy;" make a referral to mental health nurse or psychiatrist, if advisable;
— provide for the child's physical comfort with analgesics PRN & attention to physical needs;
— give comfort by holding, rocking, stroking gently, hugging; note child's reactions/tolerance.

4) Parent–Nurse Relationship

The parent/care taker will relate to at least one nurse with trust and confidence; s/he will accept the nurse's offer to listen and to help; s/he will begin to share needs, problems, and concerns;

— be aware of your own nonverbal messages & feelings; communicate those that are positive & supporting; maintain composure & compassion, refraining from criticism or rejection;
— consider asking a mental health worker or psychiatric nurse (experienced with abused children) to assist you in working through your feelings & planning care for this pt./family;
— be honest with yourself & if you can't handle it, admit it & ask to be relieved of the assignment;
— remember the parent/care taker may themselves have been abused as a child; they may be feeling confused, overwhelmed, & frustrated by their present life situation & may welcome your genuine willingness to support, understand, & help them; conversely, they may appear to be tender, loving parents convincingly able to hide their problems & to persuade you that it is the spouse, live-in lover, or babysitter who is the abuser; in these complex cases, it is wiser to refer the family to professionals experienced in helping abusers;
— let the parent(s) know that you really care about them as persons & that you respect their feelings;
— consider asking parent(s) to keep a daily diary of their feelings & situations in which they feel stress (this may be unrealistic in a stress-ridden home with too many children, not enough money, tension among adults); tell them many other parents have the same feelings; use the diary as a way of beginning to talk through feelings (often there has been no one to listen & understand); help the person identify the triggers that set off a chain of events leading to the abuse; help them to decide to accept counseling & participate in family therapy.

5) Parent-Child Relationship

The parent(s) will develop an improved relationship with their child; the parent(s) will express satisfaction with efforts to understand and enjoy their child:

- recognize that most parents do not want to hurt their children; misunderstandings, frustration, loss of control sometimes overwhelm the person in a stressful situation; afterwards the parent often feels guilt, embarrassment, & failure as a good parent; teach them how to fulfill their wish to be good parents & to do the right thing; try to be a role model of understanding & forgiveness so the parents can forgive themselves;
- assist parents to enjoy their child; point out attributes & features of the child that are lovable; introduce the parent(s) to the pleasures of reading to the child, selecting materials that will be of interest to the parent(s) as well as to the child; consult librarian for assistance in the selection of age-appropriate materials;
- ask the parent(s) to join you & the child in simple games, doll play, drawing & painting experiences; refer to NCPG #3:30, "Play Therapy;"
- teach parent(s) about normal expectations of growth & development; refer to NCPGs #3:22–25, "Normal Growth & Development: Newborn, Infant, Toddler/Preschool, School-Age Child;"
- encourage parents to participate in the care of their child (bathing, feeding, etc.);
- provide parents with a list of parenting classes in their community & suggest they attend to learn more about children & to meet other parents;
- demonstrate how limits can be set & enforced & how discipline can be given with consistency & fairness without physical force or uncontrolled anger; refer to NCPGs #2:35, "Crisis Intervention," & #5:49, "Stress Management;"
- reinforce with praise & encouragement any parental attempts to nurture, comfort, cuddle, or express affection to the child; explain that children whose only emotional contact with parents is via abuse may provoke the parent deliberately in order to gain attention; if productive, emotionally satisfying activities are done together, the child will respond more positively & be better controlled;
- reassure parent(s) that they too have rights & needs; tell them that there is an organization of parents who can provide assistance in time of crisis & need; if no organization is available in your community, perhaps you can form a small group of parents who care enough to help & will permit you to give out their phone number(s).

Discharge Planning and Teaching Objectives/Outcomes

1) The parent(s) know(s) about, and has written down in more than one place, the Parents Anonymous toll-free, 24-hour telephone number (800/421-1353); if there is a local chapter of PA, the parent has address and phone number.
2) The child and parent(s) have a referral for family and/or individual therapy.
3) The parent(s) can identify at least two new coping mechanisms that will help reduce or eliminate episodes of child abuse and handle effectively the situations likely to induce it.
4) The child will accept placement in a temporary foster home if conditions at home make this desirable or necessary for safety. The parent(s) will accept this while they get the help they need.

Recommended References

"Child Abuse: Fallout In Adulthood," (anonymous author) and "Skills For Helping Others To Redirect Emotional Responses," by J. Marder. *AORN Journal*, October 1981:651–671.
"The Child Victim of Rape/Sexual Assault." *NCP Guide #4:27*, 2nd Ed., Nurseco, 1983.
"Crisis Intervention: Adaptation to General Nursing." *NCP Guide #2:35*, 2nd Ed., Nurseco, 1980.
"Maltreatment of Children—the Tragedy of Yesterday and Today," by J. Cohen et al. *International Nursing Review*, July/August 1981:105–107.
"Normal Growth & Development: Newborn to Adolescent." *NCP Guides #3:22-26*, 2nd Ed., Nurseco, 1983.
"Nurse Abuse—Nurse Abusers," by M. Kohnke. *Nursing Health Care*, May 1981:256-260.
"Play Therapy: General Suggestions." *NCP Guide #3:30*, 2nd Ed., Nurseco, 1983.
"Prevent Child Abuse" (brochure). Chicago: National Committee for Prevention of Child Abuse (111 E. Wacker Drive Suite 510, IL 60601).
"Recognizing and Helping the Abused Child," by K. Leaman. *Nursing 79*, February, 1979:65-67.
"The Scalded Child Syndrome." *Emergency Medicine*, February 29, 1980:71,72.
Something Happened To Me, by P. Sweet. Racine, WI: Mother Courage Press (224 State St., 53103), 1981.
"Stress Management." *NCP Guide #5:49*, Nurseco, 1981.
"Symposium on Child Abuse and Neglect," by M. Heindl, Ed. *Nursing Clinics of North America*, March 1981:101–188.

The Child with a Developmental Disability: Mental Retardation (in an Acute Setting)

LONG TERM GOAL: The child will maintain admission level of functioning (or by time of discharge will have returned to admission level) within limits imposed by physical illness.

General Considerations:

— Read NCPGs #4:22, "The Child with a Developmental Disability: Mental Retardation (in a Residential Setting)," and #4:38, "The (Adult) Client with a Developmental Disability: Mental Retardation (in a Residential Setting)."

— Children with mental retardation (MR) are subject to all the common illnesses and accidents that afflict normal children. In addition, these children often have physical and allied health problems as another dimension of the existing mental retardation. These problems often make such children more prone to respiratory and secondary infections during hospitalization than other children. Childhood accidents such as falls occur more commonly in children with MR.

— MR children may convalesce slower than other children, depending on their level of functioning, and have similar fears of separation anxiety.

— The physical setting in which the child resides (home, residential, institutional, etc.) may be an important factor influencing understanding of the behavior the child exhibits.

— **Nursing responsibilities** include astute, sophisticated assessment of child behavior to differentiate between behavior that is due to hospitalization and normal patterns (nursing care time for the nonverbal or limited-speech patients may need to be increased in order to assess and anticipate behavioral psychologic needs), as well as helping the child/family adjust to the demands and limitations of the acute illness.

Specific Considerations, Potential Patient Outcomes, and Nursing Actions:

1) Psychosocial Adjustment to Hospitalization

The child/family/care taker will express feelings they may be experiencing; the child/family/care taker will verbalize their understanding of the need for hospitalization; the child will adjust to hospital environment and exhibit indications of trust and security:

— assess child/family/care taker's level of understanding & acceptance of health status; correct any misunderstandings & health teach PRN;

— encourage & allow time for child/family/care taker to express feelings/understanding in their own unique way;

— accept expressed feelings in a nonjudgmental way in both your words & actions; let them know that others in similar situations experience the same feelings;

- permit verbal expressions of anger at the hospital system & its care of the pt. & if possible, rechannel into discussion allowing expression of real feelings;
- provide sameness & consistency in nursing care since these children frequently respond better to exact schedules & time frames;
- if possible, schedule all care (including meds) so that it will be given by the same nurse;
- adjust hospital routine to child's usual one as much as possible;
- follow through on what you tell child; e.g., if you say you will return at a specific time, do so, since this helps build trust;
- provide toys, games, etc., that are appropriate to age & level of functioning;
- permit favorite toys, etc., from home or other residence to stay in bed &/or room with child;
- allow interaction from child's peers, family members, or care takers so child maintains his/her significant relationships; most especially, ask for their assistance in correctly interpreting pt.'s communication & behavior; allow them to provide care when possible;
- allow the child to participate in decision making regarding his/her care as much as possible;
- assess strengths of child, family, &/or care taker & incorporate into daily nursing care plan;
- refer to NCPG #3:20, "The Child With Separation Anxiety."

2) Maintenance of Physiologic Functioning and Comfort

The retarded child will develop and maintain as much independence as possible in activities of daily living (ADL); the child will experience minimum pain and discomfort; the child will ingest adequate food and fluid to meet body needs:

- assess child's pre-admission level of functioning; obtain information from child/family/care taker;
- depending on level of functioning, accurate assessment of pain & bodily needs is critical to ensure adequate food & fluid intake, as well as minimal pain;
- allow child's participation in ADL as long as undue fatigue is avoided & energy levels are not depleted;
- use passive and active ROM as tolerated (see NCPG #1:47, "Range of Motion Exercises"); encourage as much ambulation as possible;
- ensure adequate intake of food & fluid; use supplements when necessary & allow choice of food when possible; if child uses special feeding utensils, be sure they are present in advance;
- preserve skin integrity by massage, bathing, use of lotions, sheepskins, water mattress, etc.;

- do not wait for call light; plan regular checks so child expects you;
- remain with child until meds are safely swallowed;
- explain & demonstrate use of support systems such as suctioning, gavaging, etc., in advance so when used, will not cause fear or be removed by child;
- if child is incontinent, maintain cleanliness of person, bed, etc.;
- measure & record I&O; note BM consistency & frequency, urine specific gravity to ensure dehydration is not occurring;
- observe for restlessness, agitation, etc. (may be indicative of fever, infections);
- refer to NCPGs for specific disease entity;
- teach child/family/care taker any skills that may need to be employed after discharge, e.g., dressing changes.

3) Safety

The child will cooperate with hospital rules and regulations regarding safety at his/her level of understanding; the child will be safeguarded from preventable accident or injury:

- be aware that child may not be able to ask for help & may need to rely on nurse's assessment & judgment on what safety precautions are appropriate;
- check frequently that safety rails remain up; if restraints are necessary, stay with child until relaxed & then make frequent checks; do not underestimate child's strength;
- assist with grooming, bathing as appropriate since bathroom in hospital may not be set up for retarded child;
- plan for other safety & mobility equipment (i.e., wheelchair, walker, other special equipment) in advance so when needed, delay is avoided;
- observe for mouthing of nonfood items.

4) Preparation for Transfer

The child will resume admission level of functioning (within current imposed limitations of illness) and will be able to maintain it to discharge setting:

- if possible, have staff person visit the home or other transfer site to assess the need for additional equipment or supplies at home, etc., or consult with home health nurse prior to discharge;
- arrange in advance for any nursing care needed to assist child after discharge;
- allow child to practice, as appropriate for level of functioning, any aspect of his/her care in advance if necessary to return to home with care still needed (dressing changes, soaks, etc.);

— provide information regarding community agencies that may be helpful to child, family, or care provider;
— send home sufficient amount of meds & supplies so the child will not experience any changes in color, styles, etc., of things used in hospital (sameness is important).

Discharge Planning and Teaching Objectives/Outcomes

1) (The Child/Family/Care Taker) Can demonstrate technical skills/procedures to be carried out after discharge and has an adequate amount of supplies (dressings, etc.) to do so.
2) Has an appointment for follow-up with doctor/clinic, and a referral to a community support agency (as appropriate).
3) Has a written list of medications, dosage and times to be taken. Has sufficient medication to last until follow-up visit, or knows how to obtain renewals.

Recommended References

"The Child with a Developmental Disability: Mental Retardation (in a Residential Setting)." *NCP Guide #4:22*, 2nd Ed., Nurseco, 1983.
"The Child with Separation Anxiety." *NCP Guide #3:20*, 2nd Ed., Nurseco, 1983.
"The Client with a Developmental Disability: Mental Retardation (in a Residential Setting)." *NCP Guide #4:38*, 2nd Ed., Nurseco, 1983.
"Maintaining the Hospitalized Child's Home Ties," by B. Chadwick et al. *American Journal of Nursing*, August 1978:1361-1362.
The Mentally Retarded Child and His Family, by R. Kock and J. Dobson. New York: Brunner-Mazel Publishers, 1976.
Mental Retardation Nursing Approaches to Care, by J. Curry and K. Peppe. St. Louis: Mosby, 1978.
"Range of Motion Exercises." *NCP Guide #1:47*, 2nd Ed., Nurseco, 1980.
Way to Go, by California State University and Colleges. Baltimore: University Park Press, 1978.

The Child with a Developmental Disability: Mental Retardation (in a Residential Setting)

Definition: Mental retardation, as defined by the American Association on Mental Deficiency, refers to a sub-average general intellectual functioning that originates during the developmental period and is associated with impairment in adaptive behavior.

LONG TERM GOAL: The child will experience as many "normalizing" opportunities as possible in order to develop potentials similar to nonretarded peers. The child will improve physical, social, and emotional functioning consistent with mental retardation and his/her adaptive abilities.

General Considerations:

— Mental retardation (MR) is one of five disabilities commonly referred to as developmental disabilities. The others are autism, cerebral palsy, neurological handicaps, and seizure disorders.

— Read NCPG #4:38, "The (Adult) Client with a Developmental Disability: Mental Retardation (in a Residential Setting)."

— The term "client" rather than "patient" is the more acceptable term since a child with MR is not viewed as an "ill" child.

— **A residential setting** commonly refers to a living-out-of-home situation, e.g., nursing facility, intermediate care facility, board and care home, group home, residential school, institutional setting, etc.

— Admission to a residential setting should not be considered permanent. Programming, services, etc., should be designed so that the possibility of return to the community is seen as a viable alternative.

— **Children placed in residential settings** frequently have either profound physical, mental, and/or emotional handicaps that need constant supervision. In addition they may have behavior problems so maladaptive that the opportunity to move to less restrictive settings is impaired.

— **Nursing responsibilities** include working within the interdisciplinary team to accomplish optimal outcomes for these children, and integrating the concept of "normalization" into the assessment, planning, implementation, and evaluation of each child's individual program plan.

Specific Considerations, Potential Patient Outcomes, and Nursing Actions:

1) Psychosocial Adjustment to Residential Setting

The child, family, and/or care provider will express verbally or nonverbally an understanding of mental retardation that will facilitate the child being provided "normalizing" experiences:

— assess the child/family/care provider's level of understanding & acceptance of MR; explain & discuss the concept of "normalizing" experiences that promote self-sufficiency, adjustment, & mental growth (e.g., increased contact with non-MR persons, participation in activities normal/usual for the specific age group);

— allow expressions of anger, guilt, hostility, etc.; accept those expressions in a nonjudgmental manner by both words & actions;
— permit child to express feelings, but at the same time do not allow unacceptable behavior (e.g., physical aggression that will interfere with normalizing experiences);
— provide toys, games, equipment, educational supplies, etc., that will enable the child to increase intellectual, social, motor skills, etc.;
— verbalize & interact with the child in an age-appropriate fashion; though disability may be severe, maintain dignity in all interactions with child;
— provide information to child/family/care provider about changes in child's level of functioning; include all in individual program planning;
— allow & encourage family members & normal peers & siblings to visit & interact with the child, whenever possible;
— support families through the times when they are separated (physically and/or emotionally) from the child, so that guilt & anger will be reduced;
— if home visits are possible, provide opportunities for families to discuss their feelings about visits; assist them in planning for visits so potential problems can be avoided or reduced;
— allow the child as much independence as possible in activities of daily living; self-worth should be fostered in all activities;
— provide personal space so child's belongings can be available to him/her; permit child to decorate space if s/he wishes;
— know that consistency in care & sameness of routine in events assists the child to orient to time & place; routines are readily learned & provide child with a degree of security & satisfaction;
— assist child to develop sign language, etc., when communication is minimal, so personal needs can be expressed (see Recommended References);
— astutely assess for physical &/or behavioral symptoms indicating a possible or potential illness; chart those illnesses that this child is commonly susceptible or prone toward.

2) Activities of Daily Living (ADL); Nutrition and Fluid Balance	The child will perform ADL of (state specific activity); the child will ingest adequate food and of fluids to meet body needs: — teach & encourage child to perform ADL as long as energy levels are not unsafely depleted; — refer to NCPG #4:38, #2, "Teaching/Learning Needs" for a precise teaching plan; — ensure adequate food/fluid intake; use supplements PRN; provide food choices when possible; provide correct type feeding utensils to allow child to feed self independently; — use active & passive ROM PRN & as tolerated; encourage ambulation as much as possible; refer to NCPG #1:47, "Range of Motion Exercises;" — give meds on same schedule each day, to maintain consistency & sameness; be alert to untoward side effects that may go unnoticed by this type of client.
3) Preparation for Transfer (to Home or Other Setting)	The child will maintain current levels of functioning in new setting; the child will participate in the transfer process; — assist family members or care providers in learning technical skills as well as behavioral techniques that are necessary in caring for the child (positioning, ROM, grooming, use of equipment (e.g., walkers, special feeding utensils); scheduling, routines, behavioral management techniques); refer to NCPG #5:37, "Behavior Modification;" — assist the child to participate in decision making prior to transfer; — visit the new setting with the child & family prior to transfer; orient staff at new setting about child's individual program plan; — refer child to community organizations that may be involved in the planning & managing of the transfer; — arrange for the transfer at the best time possible for the child as well as for the new agency, so minimal disruption of routine activities occurs; — plan a follow-up visit to child once transfer is completed & a short period of adjustment (2–4 weeks) has occurred.

Discharge Planning and Teaching Objectives/Outcomes

1) (The Child/Family/Caregiver) Can carry out the skills necessary to be maintained and/or improved in the new setting.
2) Has visited the new setting and has met and knows the name of at least one member of the nursing staff who will be present on the day of transfer.

Recommended References

"Behavior Modification." *NCP Guide #5:37*, Nurseco, 1981.
The Mentally Retarded Child and His Family, by R. Koch and J. Dobson. New York: Brunner-Mazel, 1976.
Mental Retardation Nursing Approaches to Care, by J. Curry and K. Peppe. St. Louis: Mosby, 1978.
"Range of Motion Exercises." *NCP Guide #1:47*, 2nd Ed., Nurseco, 1980.
Signing Exact English. Silver Spring, MD: National Association of Deaf (814 Thayer Avenue, 20910).
Way to Go, by California State University and Colleges. Baltimore: University Park Press, 1978.

The Child Undergoing Cardiac Surgery

LONG TERM GOAL: The child will undergo surgery demonstrating adequate knowledge of the procedure and care to assure optimum tolerance; the child will be in a stabilized physiologic and psychologic state prior to surgery and will recover free of preventable complications; the child and his parents will demonstrate preparedness for increased energy and activity tolerance that will result from corrective surgery.

General Considerations:

- **Cardiac surgery** on children is usually performed to correct congenital malformations of the heart and great vessels.
- **The child with a congenital heart defect** should be given an explanation of the nature of the pathologic condition as early as s/he is able to understand it; this will prepare the child for any medical and/or surgical therapy s/he may need and will alleviate uncertainties and confusion.
- Some degree of insecurity, overprotection, and slower emotional maturation can be expected in the child with a congenital cardiac defect; s/he has not been able to participate actively in class and play activities and therefore may feel alienated, incapable, and frustrated.
- **A period of regression** may occur when the child is admitted to the hospital; this should be accepted and the child should be allowed to experience it since it is a method of coping with stress.
- Read NCPGs #4:06, 07, "The Patient Undergoing Cardiac Surgery: Preoperative and Postoperative Phases (for adult patient)," for more complete information on considerations and patient care.
- **Nursing responsibilities** include preoperative assessment of knowledge and anxiety in both patient and family, followed by adequate health teaching and preparation as needed. Postoperatively, nurses are responsible for monitoring and maintaining stabilized physiologic and psychologic states in the patient, as well as helping the family cope with the stress created by the surgery. During convalescence, preparation for discharge is included in the health teaching.

Specific Considerations, Potential Patient Outcomes, and Nursing Actions:

1) Pre-op Teaching and Care — The parents and child (to his ability) will be able to discuss the important aspects of the diagnosis, its surgical correction, and postoperative care:
   - encourage the parents & the child to verbalize feelings & ask questions;
   - evaluate the degree of separation anxiety being experienced by the child (refer to NCPG #3:20, "The Child Experiencing Separation Anxiety");

— obtain information regarding the child's past hospital experiences to get a better understanding of present behaviors & fears;
— allow the child to touch equipment to be used; demonstrate equipment (IPPB, IV, chest drainage, etc.) utilizing a doll or other aids so the child may visualize more accurately the nature & function of these procedures;
— orient the child in a nonthreatening manner slowly, 1 procedure or aspect of care at a particular time, so that s/he can assimilate the information more easily & not become overanxious due to overload;
— explain to the parents & child that you will be very busy in the post-op period carrying out monitoring & care procedures that are protective, so that your activities are not interpreted by them to mean that the child is not progressing satisfactorily;
— check child for any loose teeth that may fall out during surgery & be aspirated; report any noted to MD & anesthesiologist;
— permit the child to take a favorite toy or security object to the operating room.

2) Post-op Care The child will recover from the surgical procedure with minimal regression and anxiety, free of preventable complications; the child will demonstrate increasing energy, independence, and participation in own recovery/convalescent process:

— familiarize yourself with the child's pre-op baseline recordings so that you can evaluate post-op changes;
— carry out all activities & procedures in a calm, unhurried manner so as not to engender fear in the child & parents;
— assess pain carefully in the child; observe the use of protective behaviors (such as splinting & positioning) that may indicate pain; be aware that a child may accept pain as part of his body image & exhibit irritability & unwillingness to cooperate instead of verbalizing pain;
— remember that regression & withdrawal may occur post-op as a protective device; use soft voice & touch to assure your concern & presence & to prevent feelings of abandonment;
— check child's temp frequently; be aware that an increase in temp a few hours after surgery is common when cardiopulmonary bypass has been used; know that prolonged cold can result in metabolic acidosis;
— turn child from side to side Q1-2H to maintain adequate pulmonary ventilation & drainage; control pain to ensure adequate tidal volume; remember that crying helps inflate the lungs; when bleeding has stabilized, have child cough or suction child if s/he is unable to cooperate;

— observe the child for signs of decreased cardiac output (bradycardia, poor peripheral perfusion, decreased urinary output, restlessness, irritability) since this is common for a short time after repair of tetralogy of Fallot;

— monitor & record the administration of IV fluids carefully so that they are not given too rapidly; be aware of the child's body surface area & the total volume to be given over a designated period of time as well as the drip factor of the set used; remember that no more than 500 ml of fluid should be hung at 1 time for a child under 15 years; observe the child for any signs of circulatory overload (dyspnea, orthopnea, restlessness, elevated pulse & BP, weight gain); remember that children are more susceptible to fluid overload & pulmonary edema than adults & that changes in position & crying may affect the rate of flow;

— familiarize yourself with recommended dosages of drugs used for the child & check the calculations used according to weight or surface area & age.

Discharge Planning and Teaching Objectives/Outcomes

1) (Patient/Family/Significant Other) Knows date and time for first doctor/clinic visit and has written list of prescribed medications, exercise, and/or dietary regimen.
2) Is prepared for increased energy and activity of child.
3) Know that the child will become more independent and autonomous in functioning (this can be very frightening to the parents of a child who has had to limit his activities over a long period of time).
4) Parent(s) has(have) a plan to develop satisfactory substitute activities to replace those involved in the long-term care of a sick child.

Recommended References

"Central Venous Pressure Line." *NCP Guide #2:40*, 2nd Ed., Nurseco, 1980
"Chest Tubes and Bottles: Water-Seal Drainage." *NCP Guide #1:34*, 2nd Ed., Nurseco, 1980.
"The Child Experiencing Separation Anxiety." *NCP Guide #3:20*, 2nd Ed., Nurseco, 1983.
"Congenital Cardiac Defects" (Special Feature). *American Journal of Nursing*, February 1978:255–278.
"Fluids and Electrolytes." *NCP Guides #3:48, 49*, 2nd Ed., Nurseco, 1983.
"Nursing Care Study: Transposition of the Great Arteries," by G. Foster and S. Hibbert. *Nursing Times*, August 4, 1977:1193–1195.
"The Patient Undergoing Cardiac Surgery, Preoperative and Postoperative Phases." *NCP Guides, #4:06, 07*, 2nd Ed. Nurseco, 1983.
"Postop Care of the Pediatric Cardiac Patient," by J. Felipek. *Critical Care Quarterly*, June 1980:45–53.
"Stresses and Coping Styles of Parents of Children Undergoing Open-Heart Surgery," by L. Lewandowski. *Critical Care Quarterly*, June 1980:75–84.

The Child with Diabetes Mellitus

Definition: Diabetes mellitus is a genetically determined, chronic, metabolic disorder characterized by hyperglycemia, and caused by an absolute or relative lack of insulin (the hormone produced by the beta cells of the pancreas).

LONG TERM GOAL: The child will achieve a balance of nutrition, insulin, and activity to sustain normal growth and development with a minimum of preventable diabetic complications; the child and family will accept and successfully integrate the new diabetic lifestyle into home/family/community roles.

General Considerations:

— **Classification** (latest and currently most popular description by National Diabetes Data Group):
- *Type I*, insulin-dependent diabetes mellitus (IDDM): individual needs daily insulin to prevent ketosis and to maintain life; abrupt onset at any age but usually seen in juveniles.
- *Type II*, noninsulin-dependent diabetes mellitus (NIDDM): insulin is not needed to sustain life, but is often used to achieve metabolic control; occurs at any age, but is more commonly seen in adults; this type is sub-classified into obese and nonobese groups and into treatment groups (diet alone, oral hypoglycemics, or insulin assisted).
- *Type III*, formerly called secondary diabetes, this group includes conditions of decreased carbohydrate intolerance resulting from hormones, drugs, tumors, endocrinopathies, pancreatic disease, or malnutrition.

— **Signs and symptoms:** frequent urination (polyuria), excessive thirst (polydipsia), fatigue, weight loss associated with excessive hunger (polyphagia), and chronic infections that resolve slowly.

— **Treatment** aims to achieve metabolic control and prevent complications and long-term metabolic, neurologic, cardiovascular, and other consequences of the disease. Psychologic acceptance of diabetes and self-confident responsibility for the treatment regimen are the goals of family-centered educational programs, which must continue throughout the course of the child's growth and development.

— **Nurses** (hospital, metabolic clinic, home health, and school) make a significant contribution to the assessment, education, counseling, and assistance of the patient and family to cope effectively in the long-term management of this lifetime condition. Studies show that parental attitudes toward diabetic treatment regimens are similar to their attitudes toward childrearing. Children with good to fair control are most likely to have better informed, caring parents and mothers who are flexible and assume primary responsibility for supervising diabetes management. These children often come from stable homes with a low stress environment and cooperative family relationships. Children with disturbed personalities and variable control over diabetic condition often have mothers who are overcontrolling or indifferent and rejecting in attitude. Factors other than family dynamics that affect the child's diabetic control are the emotional and cognitive development of the child, age, insight, ability to relate effectively with health care professionals, and willingness to assume responsibility for own care. After consulting with the physician about the therapeutic regimen of prescribed diet, insulin, exercise, and general care, the nurse should assess the learning readiness and needs of the child and family. Refer to NCPG #3:32, "Teaching the Parent/Guardian/Child: General Suggestions," and to the Recommended References below.

— **Glucose-controlled insulin infusion systems (GCIIS)**, while still investigational, show promise for maintaining normal or near normal blood glucose levels (80–104 mg/dl) in IDDM-juveniles. These portable, battery-operated infusion pumps are attached to patient and deliver insulin subcutaneously in between-meal and before-meal increments. A glucose sensor and preprogrammed controlling computer complete the unit. Patients can pursue normal activities outside the hospital with a minimum of interference. It remains to be seen whether the long-term complications of diabetes can be prevented or delayed through this method of improved metabolic control.

Specific Considerations, Potential Patient Outcomes, and Nursing Actions:

1) Assessment of Current Status

The patient will be free of the signs and symptoms of glucose/insulin imbalance:
- record I&O accurately; weigh daily;
- test urine for sugar & acetone Q1H 1st 24 hours & QID after condition stabilizes;
- use NCPGs #3:19, "The Child: Nursing Assessment Guide," #s3:23–26, "Normal Growth & Development (Infant through Adolescence)," to assess learning needs & child's growth & development status;
- record & report changes in TPR & BP;
- observe & record signs of ketoacidosis & hypoglycemia; refer to NCPG #1:35, "Differentiating Hypoglycemia and Ketoacidosis;"
- monitor parenteral therapy for accuracy, safety, & correct rate of administration.

2) Nutrition

The patient will ingest adequate nutritional intake for activity level and growth, and to maintain ideal body weight; the patient will eat most of diet at regular meal times and prescribed snack times; the patient will understand and assume responsibility for eating suitable foods prior to vigorous exercise or when recognizing hypoglycemic signs:
- give all meals & snacks on time; teach child/family the importance of this; record & measure amounts not eaten & give replacement carbohydrate feeding; teach family how to do this (no child can be expected to eat full amounts of all desired foods on diet plan); refer to NCPG #1:37, "Liquid Diet Substitutes for the Diabetic;"

- know that some children will be permitted a liberal dietary regimen & others will be on a more strictly controlled one; understand which approach will be used & teach accordingly;
- explain that while it is normal to "cheat" on diet occasionally, the possible harmful consequences can come about rather suddenly at times & at other times not at all; teach child & parent how to compensate appropriately using food exchange lists for some food favorites (e.g., pizza = 1 bread, 2 fat, 1 protein);
- warn that problems can occur if a whole meal is skipped; teach child to carry nutritious snack (cheese & crackers, nuts, can of water-based fruit, or fresh fruit) in case a meal is unavoidably delayed; have the child carry hard candy only for cases of emergency hypoglycemic reaction;
- know & teach that improved blood glucose control can be achieved by eating high fiber, whole carbohydrates (fresh fruits & vegetables, whole grain breads & cereals) rather than processed foods (white bread, dry commercial cereals, canned fruits or vegetables that have been cooked);
- teach child/family what kinds of foods can be eaten in a restaurant that will fit into dietary plan & not make the youngster feel different when s/he's around friends.

3) Exercise — The patient will maintain normal indoor & outdoor activity levels for age in balance with the amount of insulin & diet being given; the child/family will indicate an understanding of the importance of daily activity/sports/physical education for optimal healthy growth & development as well as good diabetes management:

- simulate a "normal" active day as much as possible in the hospital setting; encourage play & socialization with other children;
- explain to child/family the purpose of exercise/activity & the need for carbohydrates just before extra exertion, such as sporting events in which the child will participate, or physical education classes.

4) Medication — The patient/family will administer insulin with accuracy and safety, demonstrating satisfactory proficiency:

- see NCPG #1:38, "Properties of Insulin Preparations;" teach child/family about insulin, its storage & handling, its activity & effects; continue to reassess knowledge regarding these areas in subsequent hospitalizations & clinic visits;
- know that the most frequent error made by children administering self-injections of insulin is having bubbles in the insulin syringe, causing errors of dosage; know also that insulin syringes have "dead space" in syringe & needle that can make a significant difference if using U-80 insulin &/or U-100 syringes; use plastic syringes whose dead space is known to be minimal or arrange for compensating dosage error in consultation with MD;

— teach at least 2 family members to administer insulin accurately, safely, & with satisfactory proficiency; children 8 years of age or older should be taught to give their own insulin under supervision; teach child to give injection at 90° (right) angle to the skin (easier & less painful); have the child practice with an orange or suitable plastic doll; if possible, have the child & parent watch other children give their own injections;
— teach child & family the factors that increase insulin need (e.g., trauma, infection, exposure to cold, fever, stress, & tension) & to avoid these factors *when possible*; if these influences are unavoidable, then seek prompt medical advice;
— teach the importance & method of site rotation & provide a suitable chart for recording sites used & dates;
— observe & record demonstrated ability of family (& child if appropriate) to handle, clean, sterilize & safely store equipment & supplies; have family bring in their own pot & strainer for sterilization (if disposable syringes & needles are not economically feasible).

5) Urine Testing — The patient and two family members will accurately demonstrate the two-drop Clinitest method and the Acetest:
— explain reasons for not touching tablets or test paper with fingers;
— explain the bright orange "pass-through" phenomenon when glycosuria is too high to react accurately;
— remind them of the importance of using fresh 2nd-voided specimens in clean containers, discarding 1st morning and 1st voided (after 2 hours) before-meal specimens;
— provide record form for listing urine test results & times.

6) Prevention of Complications — The patient/family will define terms: ketoacidosis, hypoglycemia, hyperglycemia, glucagon, ketonuria, acetones; the patient/family will demonstrate knowledge of good oral hygiene, proper skin and foot care and the signs and symptoms of illness:
— assess what child/family knows about ketoacidosis & hypoglycemia; teach PRN, referring to NCPG #1:35;
— teach child to recognize & notice early warning signs in own body of high or low blood sugar reactions; remember that symptoms may vary in individuals; child must get to know own particular signs;
— explain & demonstrate proper skin & foot care, & oral hygiene; ask for return demonstrations; refer to NCPG #1:39, "Recommended Care of the Feet for Diabetics;"
— provide suitable literature from the local chapter of the American Diabetes Association; review with child/family; encourage questions, clear up misconceptions, repeat explanations PRN; obtain extra copies for grandparents & child's schoolteacher.

7) Psychosocial Adjustment — The child/youth will demonstrate a productive, self-reliant adjustment to his diabetic condition and management; the parents will experience relief of feelings of guilt, fear, anxiety, frustration, and confusion and will verbalize feelings of self-confidence in supervising and assisting child with control of diabetes:

— separately, then later in family group sessions, explore level of acceptance of child's diabetic condition; expect overlapping stages or periods of denial, depression, anger, & guilt with reluctant gradual acceptance;
— encourage recognition, acknowledgment, & expression of feelings (both parent & older youth will normally feel fear, anger, resentment, depression over loss of health & burden of life-long disease condition);
— use reality-based, matter-of-fact, calm, low-key approach with sensitive timing & judgment; adapt counseling & explanations to that needed & desired, tailoring each session to needs, interest, & wishes of child or parent; do not overwhelm them with too much information too soon;
— offer to provide explanations to child's siblings, grandparents, & other interested relatives; do not shut them out, but include them as soon as possible since they will ultimately have some influence on child's acceptance of self & condition;
— remind family that this child is like any other, requiring love, understanding, acceptance, & firm, consistent guidelines with discipline PRN; overindulging & overprotecting are destructive behaviors that produce maladjusted children who will rebel into a state of poor diabetic control with possible ketoacidosis;
— teach that stress elevates blood sugar; discuss appropriate stress management techniques & coping skills that can be helpful; refer to NCPG #5:49, "Stress Management;" try to put the child & parents in touch with another diabetic child & family who can provide support & encouragement; contact local Diabetes Association for peer group meetings & education lectures;
— ask the parents to visit the child's teacher & school nurse to discuss child's needs (a specific, early, lunch period; in-school snacks, not necessarily only at recess when more convenient; recognition of signs of hypoglycemia); if physical education class is not scheduled within 2 hours after a meal, arrange for child to have a carbohydrate snack (crackers, fruit, juice, milk) about 30 minutes prior to vigorous exercise;
— tell parents about opportunities for child to attend summer camp for diabetic children, so that self-respect & self-reliance can be gained as well as motivation for self-management of diabetes.

Discharge Planning and Teaching Objectives/Outcomes

1) (Patient/Family) Can answer questions: What is diabetes? What are the common symptoms, treatment, and expectations for its control? Has received at least one current pamphlet on diabetes and a written sheet of instructions.

2) Understands that a temporary remission period may occur, but that they must not entertain false hopes of a cure. State they will still observe for signs of hypoglycemia and ketoacidosis so they will be prepared when remission is over (up to 18 months).
3) Can test urine for sugar and acetone properly, and keep an accurate record.
4) Can tell about types of insulin, how to store and handle correctly. Can give own injections accurately and safely, rotating sites according to a plan and caring for equipment without contamination.
5) Can state the differing signs and symptoms of insulin reaction and ketoacidosis. Knows exactly what to do for each situation.
6) Has a printed sheet of dietary instructions and sample menus. Can understand, accept, and help plan a well balanced meal consistent with needs for growth, activity, and family living style. Knows what foods to avoid.
7) Knows the importance of good personal health habits, including exercise; daily care of teeth, feet, and skin; adequate rest and sleep; and continuing medical follow-up. Knows that emotional upsets and tension will increase the need for insulin.
8) Has appointment for follow-up medical visit. Has referral information for home health nurse visit to supervise home management.
9) Has sufficient supplies until first doctor/clinic appointment. Has bottles of insulin, syringes, 25 gauge, ½" or ⅝" needles, alcohol sponges, urine testing supplies, and record sheet.

Recommended References

"Ban the Bolus in Ketoacidosis." *Emergency Medicine*, May 15, 1980:59.
"The Child: Nursing Assessment Guide." *NCP Guide #3:19*, 2nd Ed. Nurseco, 1983.
"Cognitive and Behavioral Knowledge About Insulin-Dependent Diabetes Among Children and Parents," by S. Johnson et al. *Pediatrics*, June 1982:708–713.
"Crisis Intervention in the Problems of a Pre-School Diabetic Child," by F. Cathcart and M. Glass. *Nursing Times*, November 11, 1981:1981–1982.
"Diabetes: New Systems for Classification and Diagnosis," by A. Khachadurian. *Geriatrics*, January 1982:111–115.
"Differentiating Hypoglycemia and Ketoacidosis." *NCP Guide #1:35*, 2nd Ed., Nurseco, 1980.
"General Dietary Principles for the Diabetic." *NCP Guide #1:36*, 2nd Ed., Nurseco, 1980.
"Growing Up Diabetic," by I. Rosofsky. *Family Health*, November/December 1980:26–32, 63.
"Liquid Diet Substitutes for the Diabetic." *NCP Guide #1:37*, 2nd Ed., Nurseco, 1980.
"Normal Growth and Development (Infant to Adolescent)." *NCP Guides #3:23-26*, 2nd Ed., Nurseco, 1983.
"Nursing Care for Children with Hypoglycemia Due to Hyperinsulinism," by D. Fendya et al. *MCN: American Journal of Maternal Child Nursing,* March/April 1981:100–105.
"Outpatient Treatment of Juvenile-Onset Diabetes with a Preprogrammed Portable Subcutaneous Insulin Infusion System," by W. Tamborlane et al. *American Journal of Medicine*, February 1980:190–196.
"Properties of Insulin Preparations." *NCP Guide #1:38*, 2nd Ed., Nurseco, 1980.
"Recommended Care of the Feet for Diabetics." *NCP Guide #1:39*, 2nd Ed., Nurseco, 1980.
"Research on Diabetes Management and the Family: A Critique," by B. Anderson and W. Auslander. *Diabetes Care*, November/December 1980:696–702.
"Stress Management." *NCP Guide #5:49*, Nurseco, 1981.
"Teaching the Parent/Guardian/Child: General Suggestions." *NCP Guide #3:32*, 2nd Ed., Nurseco, 1983.
"What School Personnel Should Know About the Student with Diabetes" and "What You Need to Know About Diabetes." New York: American Diabetes Association.

The Child who is Dying/Terminal

LONG TERM GOAL: The child will maintain physiologic and emotional functioning with comfort and reduced anxiety during the terminal process. The family will move toward acceptance and resolution of the terminal process, so they can assist in providing comfort and support to the dying child.

General Considerations:

— The **age of the child** must be considered in relation to his/her level of understanding regarding death and dying. Young children may equate death with (1) separation, departure, disappearance; (2) going into a grave, coffin, earth, or water; or (3) sleep.

— **Societal and cultural values** influence both children and adults in their acceptance of death. Understanding of those value systems influences perceptions of and reactions to the knowledge that a child is dying. ("It isn't fair. He never even got to experience the pleasures and pain of growing up.")

— **Previous experiences** with death such as the death of a pet, another family member, a family friend, and/or a peer will influence the child's perception of and reaction to death. Read NCPG #5:24, "The Child's Conception of Death."

— Children will convey their feelings and level of understanding of their impending death through symbols (drawings that over time are colored darker), through play with toys and other children, and by behaviors such as anger, hostility, withdrawal, apathy, etc.

— The appearance of a lack of understanding on the child's part about what is happening does not mean the child has no anxiety about death and dying.

— Children perceive alterations in staff and family behavior around them, and may adjust their own reaction to death based on adult behavior.

— **Nursing responsibilities** include helping the child/family move adaptively through the grieving process; helping the child maintain physiological functioning with comfort for as long as possible; and identifying personal feelings regarding loss and the impact that that might have on his/her ability to carry out nursing responsibilities professionally.

Specific Considerations, Potential Patient Outcomes, and Nursing Actions:

1) Psychosocial Adjustment — The child/family will express feelings, fears, anxieties, guilt they may be experiencing; will verbalize their understanding of the physical health status and the terminal process:

— assess the child's & family's level of understanding & acceptance of the physical-health status; tell them that others in the same situation experience many kinds of feelings; ask them what it is like for them just now;
— allow & encourage the parents to express their feelings & accept those expressions in a nonjudgmental manner;
— permit child to express anger & hostility, but at the same time do not allow total permissiveness regarding unacceptable behavior, since the child may perceive this permissiveness as hopelessness & abandonment;
— provide age-appropriate toys, pens, pencils, etc., that will enable the child to have normalizing experiences & symbolically express his level of understanding regarding death;
— avoid false cheerfulness & evasiveness that may prevent the child from expressing true feelings;
— at the child's level of understanding, allow discussion of the physical manifestations of the illness, the diagnosis, & possible outcomes;
— give information to the child & family about changes that are occurring in the body;
— allow family members, friends, peers, to continue interaction with the child; be available to these "significant others" if the child withdraws from their attempt to comfort;
— as much as possible, allow the child to make decisions regarding physical care, setting the time for required procedures to be performed, & participating in daily activities;
— allow the family to assist with the child's care, or if that is not feasible, to assist with the care of other children on the ward (if the child & family desire & accept this);
— keep the family informed on the daily medical & nursing regimen so they can be kept abreast of the child's physical & emotional functioning;
— assess the parents' behavior astutely so that when they need support, are unable to care for their child, & need to be alone, feelings of guilt will be avoided; seek consultation from a psychiatric/mental health nurse PRN;
— assess the strengths of the parents & utilize those strengths in planning the management of the child;
— provide opportunities for staff discussion of home care so that if this is a viable alternative, home care can be arranged; criteria for such discussion should focus on:
  • the child wants to be home, the family wants the child to be home & they feel they are able to care for him/her;
  • cure-oriented treatment has been discontinued;

	• nurse, MD, &/or other team members are available for on-call consultation; — when possible, allow the child & family to leave the hospital for short periods to have dinner, go to a park, attend a movie, visit with other children, etc.
2) Maintenance of Physiologic Function	The child will maintain as much independence as possible in activities of daily living (ADL); the child will experience minimum pain and discomfort; the child will ingest adequate food and fluid to meet body needs; — assess pain & provide medication PRN; use oral medications whenever possible; attempt to reserve heavy doses of narcotics until late in illness; — encourage the child's participation in ADL as long as the child's energy levels are not depleted; — use passive & active range-of-motion exercises as tolerated (see NCPG #1:47); encourage as much ambulation as possible; — ensure adequate intake of fluid & food; use supplements when necessary & allow child choice of food if possible; — preserve skin integrity by massage, bathing, use of lotions, sheepskins, water mattress, etc.; — maintain a pleasing physical environment by allowing adequate ventilation of the room, use of room deodorants when necessary, permitting toys & material objects of importance to the child to be present; — allow child to wear own clothing when possible.
3) Preparation for Transfer of Child to Home or Non-Acute Setting	The child will maintain current level of functioning in new setting: — assist family members to learn the technical skills necessary to care for the child's physical needs at home (administration of medications, positioning, ROM exercises, bathing, skin care, use of equipment such as bedpans, bedside commodes, suctioning devices, etc.); — assist the family &, if appropriate, the child to recognize need for meds & the amount necessary to maintain comfort; — make home visit to assist family in setting up the home for the child prior to discharge; — refer to VNA, health department, home health agency, hospice, etc., to obtain additional professional assistance as necessary; — go with family to visit the non-acute setting to which the child may be transferred in advance of the actual transfer;

— assist the family as necessary & as desired in anticipating funeral arrangements; arrange for social service agencies & resource persons such as clergy, etc., to be available;
— refer family & parents to self-help groups in their community; keep a list available at your nursing unit for convenient use; the local chapter of the American Cancer Society or Community Mental Health Center also can give parent names of such groups.

Discharge Planning and Teaching Objectives/Outcomes:

1) (The Child and/or Family) Can carry out technical skills needed to care for self/child at home.
2) Has expressed some degree of awareness of the terminal process and feelings associated with loss, grief and mourning.
3) Has a referral to a community support group.
4) Has been made aware that if, at any time during the home-care period, there are feelings that the family cannot go on with the decision to maintain child at home, returning to the hospital or other care setting is not a failure on their part.

Recommended References

"An Alternative to Institutionalization for Severely Involved Newborns," by M. Challela in *Mental Retardation, Nursing Approaches to Care*. St. Louis: Mosby, 1978.
"The Child's Conception of Death." *NCP Guide #5:24*, Nurseco, 1981.
"The Child with Leukemia: Parents Help Each Other," by I. Martinson. *American Journal of Nursing*, July 1976:1120–1122.
"The Dying Child," by F. Northrup. *American Journal of Nursing*, June 1974:1066–1068.
"The Dying Person and the Family," by N. Doyle. *Public Affairs Pamphlet #485*, New York: Public Affairs Committee, 1974.
"Home Care for the Child," by I. Martinson et al. *American Journal of Nursing*, November 1977:1816–1817.
"I Am a Yellow Ship," by S. Grove. *American Journal of Nursing*, March 1978:414.
"Range of Motion Exercises." *NCP Guide #1:47*, 2nd Ed., Nurseco, 1980.

The Child with Leukemia

LONG TERM GOAL: The child will live as long as possible, with minimum necessary restrictions and discomforts.

General Considerations:

- Read this section in NCPG #4:13, "The Patient with Leukemia."
- **Leukemia** is the principal type of cancer in children. It is usually acute lymphocytic leukemia (ALL), which accounts for 80% of all leukemia in children.
- **Onset** may be abrupt or insidious, and usually occurs between two and five years of age; slightly more frequent in boys than in girls.
- **Signs and symptoms** include anorexia, nausea and vomiting, anemia, weight loss, pallor, weakness, fatigue, intermittent temperature, dyspnea, bone and joint pain.
- **Treatment** is supportive, palliative, specific, and aimed at cure.
- **Prognosis:** with treatment, 50% of children with ALL will have a five-year survival. Children who develop it between the ages of two and eight years usually survive longer than infants or children over eight years.
- **Nursing responsibilities** include reducing susceptibility to infection and hemorrhage; minimizing side effects of treatment regimen; and working with child/family to help them move adaptively through the grieving process as they adjust to change and/or impending death.

Specific Considerations, Potential Patient Outcomes, and Nursing Actions:

1) Susceptibility to Infection — The patient will be free of hospital-based infection; the patient/family will carry out measures to prevent infections:

- isolate from persons with an infectious disease (some specific regimens may require strict reverse isolation); maintain a hygienic environment & carry out medical asepsis;
- ensure child washes hands after urinating or a BM;
- teach family rationale & principles of isolation & medical asepsis;
- monitor vital signs & be aware of changes that may indicate an early infection (e.g., increasing TPR); avoid rectal temps since damaged mucosa is a site for bacteria;
- examine skin & mucous membranes QD for any lesions or breaks;

— provide mouth care frequently in order to maintain integrity of mucous membranes; use only soft toothbrushes & mouth swabs & nonirritating mouthwashes, such as hydrogen peroxide.

2) Increased Risk of Hemorrhage	The patient will be monitored for early signs of hemorrhage; the patient will take precautions to reduce risk of bleeding: — pad crib/bed PRN to minimize trauma; — handle pt. gently; do not pull across sheets; — inspect skin & mucous membranes daily for signs of bleeding; instruct pt. to blow nose gently, not to pick at nose; keep lips & nostrils lubricated; — examine each stool & urine for gross evidence of bleeding; — use small-gauge needles for all injections & apply pressure dressing after needle removal; — know normal parameters of blood-cell constituents & monitor pt. & blood studies for abnormal results or changes; share with pt./family as you judge appropriate; — keep floor clear of objects that could cause pt. to fall; provide soft toys & books, avoid sharp objects; — assess what pt./family knows about transfusions; health teach PRN. — report any signs/symptoms of hemorrhage (decreased BP, tachycardia, pallor, diaphoresis, increased anxiety).
3) Nutrition	The patient will ingest adequate food and fluids to maintain normal weight, support growth, and help prevent infection: — weigh at least weekly & chart; — assess what child likes to eat & drink & try to include in menu; involve pt. & family in food selection; — provide oral hygiene prior to each meal; — let family members be present at mealtimes; explain the need for special diet, e.g., increased protein as a booster against infection; — avoid irritating foods & hot liquids as a measure to prevent breaks in mucosa & bleeding gums; cool drinks & soft food are soothing to irritated mucosa; — chart food intake, as well as I&O; — schedule meals around chemotherapy; control nausea with antiemetics.

— be aware that lysis of leukemic cells produces an increase of uric acid content in body & increased uric acid excretion that may precipitate in the tubules causing intrarenal obstruction & anuria; give at least 2500 ml of fluids per day & alkalinize the urine to prevent precipitation.

4) Psychosocial Adjustment (to Loss) The patient/family will deal adaptively with changes in body image and usual role functioning; the patient/family will express feelings, fear, anxieties about the disease process and/or impending death:

— read NCPG #4:25, "The Child who is Dying/Terminal;"
— refer to NCPGs #1:27, "Impending Death," #1:31, "Responses to Loss," and #2:29, "Body Image Disturbance;"
— allow & encourage family to provide care for child as much as possible;
— accept all feelings pt./family express, including negative ones; know that this is part of the process of adjustment;
— be alert to children expressing feelings, fears through play, e.g., with toys or drawing pictures; encourage such expressions as "Where are you in this picture?" Refer to NCPG #5:24, "The Child's Conception of Death;"
— provide diversionary play for pt. within safe limits; refer to NCPG #3:30, "Play Therapy;"
— explain all treatments to child at his/her level of understanding; encourage child to ask questions about treatment (providing information can lower anxieties & eradicate fears);
— reinforce family for focusing on short-range planning, 1 day at a time.

5) Drug Therapy The patient will be monitored for early signs and symptoms of side effects and toxicity; the patient will receive interventions to counteract untoward effects:

— refer to NCPG #4:44, "Drugs: Antileukemic;"
— use appropriate references (PDR, manufacturers' literature) to become knowledgeable about the drugs, their actions & effects, preparation & administration;
— mix oral meds with fruit, ice cream, etc., PRN to aid ingestion;
— provide supportive & comfort measures for side effects, which are usually pronounced (minimizing these will require much nursing time, skill, & patience);
— teach pt./family drug actions, side effects, & toxic manifestations.

Discharge Planning and Teaching Objectives/Outcomes:

1) (Patient and/or Family) Knows measures to carry out to prevent infection. Can verbalize early signs and symptoms of infection, and knows to report them promptly to doctor/clinic.
2) Has a written list of medications, with times, dosage, and possible side effects. Knows toxic manifestations and methods to minimize them.
3) Knows to report any bleeding promptly, and to apply pressure PRN. Verbalizes preventive measures against trauma.
4) Can select a diet specific to nutritional needs. Knows to avoid foods irritating to mucosa.
5) Can verbalize some feelings about disease, changes in life style, roles, and is coping adaptively with subsequent changes.
6) Has information/referral to a community support group and home health service. Has an appointment for follow-up medical treatment with doctor/clinic.

Recommended References

"Acute Lymphoid Leukemia in Children," by C. Pochedly. *American Journal of Nursing*, October 1978:1714–1716.
"The Child who is Dying/Terminal." *NCP Guide #4:25*, 2nd Ed., Nurseco, 1983.
"The Child's Conception of Death." *NCP Guide #5:24*, Nurseco, 1981.
"Dealing with Impending Death." *NCP Guide #1:27*, 2nd Ed., Nurseco, 1980.
"Drugs: Antileukemic." *NCP Guide #4:44*, 2nd Ed., Nurseco, 1983.
"Leukemia: Part I: A Hematology Review," by N. Houlihan. *Cancer Nursing*, February 1981:61–71.
Part II: "The Leukemic Process," by N. Houlihan. *Cancer Nursing*, April 1981:149–160.
Part III: "The Treatment of Leukemia," by A. Feeley and N. Houlihan. *Cancer Nursing*, June 1981:233–245.
Part IV: "The Acute & Chronic Leukemias," by A. Feeley and N. Houlihan. *Cancer Nursing*, August 1981:323–338.
Part V: "Nursing Management," by A. Feely and N. Houlihan. *Cancer Nursing*, October 1981:397–405.
"Nursing the Child with Leukemia," by C. Pochedly, MD. *Journal of Practical Nursing*, September 1978:16–18.
"Nursing Care Plan for the Child with Acute Leukemia," by M. Boecke. *Journal of Practical Nursing*, September 1978:19–21.
"The Patient Experiencing a Body Image Disturbance." *NCP Guide #2:29*, 2nd Ed., Nurseco, 1980.
"The Patient with Leukemia." *NCP Guide #4:13*, 2nd Ed., Nurseco, 1983.
"Play Therapy." *NCP Guide #3:30*, 2nd Ed., Nurseco, 1983.
"Responses to Loss: The Grief and Mourning Process." *NCP Guide #1:31*, 2nd Ed., Nurseco, 1980.

The Child Victim of Rape/Sexual Assault

LONG TERM GOAL: The child will experience protection from pain, injury, anxiety, fear, and real or potential physical abuse.

General Considerations:

— Read NCPGs #4:34, "The Adult Victim of Rape/Sexual Assault (in the ER)," and #2:35, "Crisis Intervention."

— **Sexual assaults on children** are usually grouped into two categories: (1) *forced rape*, most frequently an isolated, traumatic event with physical injury, generating fear and pain in the child; child is more upset over the pain and violence than the sexual activity; (2) *accessory-to-sex*, usually involving exposure, statutory rape, incest, molestation, but not force; recurring episodes may extend over a period of time.

— **Offenders** in accessory-to-sex assaults are usually an adult the child knows, most frequently a family member or relative, sometimes a neighbor. The offender usually bribes the child with money, candy, etc.; threats, authority, and domination are often used to generate fear in the child and thus maintain secrecy of the assault(s). Children may not tell anyone of the assault(s) for fear of being punished, blamed, or disbelieved but may develop somatic and behavioral symptoms.

— **The major traumatic impact** on the child is psychologic rather than physical. The child will react to the family/significant other's (SO) reaction more than to the assault itself. The child views the event far differently than an adult and when it is dealt with calmly, will usually have no long-term psychologic scars.

— **The ER nurse's responsibilities** are to believe what the child says; to provide basic crisis intervention to both child and family/SOs; to assist with medical treatment, collect and prepare physical evidence; and to refer child, family/SO for follow-up physical and mental-health treatment; s/he also needs to identify personal feelings so that professional responsibilities are conducted in accordance with the needs of the child, family/SOs, and mandated legal requirements.

Specific Considerations, Potential Patient Outcomes, and Nursing Actions:

1) Acute Physical and Emotional Reaction (Rape/Trauma Syndrome)	The child will receive situational support from ER staff and will be allowed to cope with situation in own way: — encourage the child to talk about the experience & to ventilate feelings but do not dwell on the sexual aspects; suggest drawing a picture of what happened & to talk about the drawing (often easier for children to do than just talk); do not minimize child's feelings or try to talk them away, but acknowledge them; — know that these children are often misbelieved; let child know you believe what s/he says, thinks, feels; — use a calm, soothing approach to child, showing your caring, warmth, & interest in her/him as a person; — reinforce to child that it was not her/his fault, that s/he will not be punished, & that s/he is not a bad child;

— explain all procedures to child before they are carried out as they may be more frightening to the child than the sexual assault; read NCPG #4:46; ensure that a female (staff, police, family) stays with female child at all times.

2) Reaction of Family/SOs — The family/SOs will state they feel less anxious and are able to cope with situation; they will verbalize an understanding of what child has experienced and will provide situational support for child:

— talk to family away from child in order to help them sort out their feelings of anger, anxiety, fear, etc.; encourage them to ventilate to you rather than to child (child may then feel guilty for upsetting the family);
— inform family that the child will respond more to their reactions than to the assault;
— know that the family/SOs may vent anger at the offender, at the agency/staff, or even the child, especially if the offender is someone they know & like;
— assess their level of coping; if they are hysterical, be very firm, authoritarian if necessary, to calm them down; provide general support (listen, acknowledge feelings) to enhance their own coping ability;
— help them focus on the needs of the child right now, rather than on the attacker; point out that the child needs loving, stroking, holding, caring, to feel s/he is not "bad," was not at fault;
— reinforce that the responsibility for the assault lies with the offender, not with the child; family/SOs may be confused, disbelieving, especially if offender is a family member, friend, or neighbor;
— if they talk of the child being "ruined" or "violated," or "she's no longer my little girl," point out that she is indeed still a little girl, the same child who now has a great need for support, love, reassurance, & protection;
— tell them the child may or may not want to talk about the assault & that they should let the child set the pace, not forcing him/her or criticizing in any way;
— stress the importance of returning to usual family activities as soon as possible; discuss the benefits of family mental-health counseling & provide community referrals as necessary.

Discharge Planning and Teaching Objectives/Outcomes:

1) (Child/Family/Significant Other) Have been given a written list of referrals for follow-up physical and mental health care.
2) State they feel in control of situation and can describe verbally their plans to protect the child from further abuse.

Recommended References

"Crisis Intervention." *NCP Guide #2:35*, 2nd Ed., Nurseco, 1980.
"Evidence Collection: Rape/Sexual Assault." *NCP Guide #4:46*, 2nd Ed., Nurseco 1983.
Prevention of Abuse and Neglect of Children in Out-of-Home Care, by E. Jil. San Francisco: San Francisco Child Abuse Council, 1979.

The Child/Youth with Scoliosis: Medical Management

Definition: Scoliosis is an abnormal lateral curvature of the spine; the condition sometimes includes secondary compensation curves and rotation of vertebral bodies; occasionally the patient will also have hyperlordosis (excessive swayback) and/or kyphosis (excessive rounded upper back).

LONG TERM GOAL: The child/youth will achieve a normal life with a straight, healthy back via the least restrictive means necessary to achieve correction of curvature; the child/youth will express a feeling of independence and responsibility for self-care and the success of treatment.

General Considerations:

— **Incidence and occurrence:** an estimated one million Americans have some lateral curvature of spine; about 4%–14% of 10- to 14-year-olds have signs but only a small percentage of these require continuing observation or treatment. Curves under 10° are seen with equal frequency among boys and girls; curves over 20° are five to seven times more prevalent in girls.

— **Types and causes:** *functional (flexible) scoliosis* is of two kinds, postural and compensatory, related to unequal leg lengths, habitual poor posture, weakened spinal muscles, or muscle disorders. *Structural (inflexible) scoliosis* is of three kinds, congenital (related to birth injuries or developmental disabilities), neuromuscular/paralytic (due to disease or trauma), and idiopathic (no identifiable cause). The latter type is sometimes referred to as familial because of sex linkage and tendency to run in families. More than 80% of all cases are believed to be idiopathic.

— **School screening programs** for boys and girls in sixth, seventh, and eighth grades are an effective mechanism for early detection and diagnosis, and are required by law in many states.

— **Treatment** is aimed at curvature correction and maintenance through skeletal maturity and periods of risk (pregnancy, obesity, disease). Mild curvatures of less than 20° are observed for progression every three to six months by an orthopedic specialist; sometimes they correct themselves or can be modified with corrective heel lifts or exercises and improved posture. Moderate curvatures (20°–40°) are often treated with a Milwaukee brace and exercises or the more modern Thoraco-Lumbo-Sacral Orthosis (TLSO) jacket. The latter is cosmetically preferable to youths. Recently some success has been reported with the nighttime use of electrical stimulation (100 milliamperes) externally to strengthen muscles on the convex side of the curve. The scolatron (part computer) also records usage; at least two to three hours/night are needed for effectiveness. Curvatures greater than 40° may be treated with Cotrel traction, spinal-fusion surgery, and a Risser body cast for six to 12 months. Surgery is indicated when the deformity is cosmetically objectionable, when the curvature is progressive and unamenable to conservative measures, and when persistent backache is not controlled satisfactorily. A 50% improvement of the curvature is considered a successful surgical outcome.

— **Nursing responsibilities** (school, home health, orthopedic clinic) include (1) competent screening of pre-adolescents; (2) referring child for follow-up evaluation; (3) helping the child/youth and family understand the current condition and accept the necessary treatment; and (4) teaching the family how to provide the care needed to ensure success of selected treatment plan.

Specific Considerations, Potential Patient Outcomes, and Nursing Actions:

1) Screening Process

The patient will be correctly identified as having a possible spine abnormality; the patient will see an orthopedic specialist for diagnosis and treatment:

— participate in a special inservice-training session with other school nurses, physical education teachers, public health nurses, volunteer parents, MDs, & school administrators; discuss the scope of the program & procedure for examination & referral; show educational films;
— notify parents & obtain signed consent forms; offer opportunities for the parents to participate in the screening program & to learn more about diagnosis & treatment;
— during screening process, arrange for privacy during undressing & examination (boys are stripped to the waist, girls to the bra);
— observe body alignment from the front, side, back while child/youth is standing erect & bending forward about 60° with arms extended & hands touching; note asymmetrical chest or shoulder height, a prominent shoulder blade or ribs, unlevel hips, or sideways deviation of the spine;
— record pertinent data on screening form; use later to record subsequent referral & follow-up care;
— make telephone & written referral to parents if there is a need for specialist confirmation & x-rays;
— follow-up visit with parents to determine if the child/youth has been seen by an MD (1 out of 5 has not); ask them to share their feelings regarding the outcome of visit or reasons for choosing not to seek medical advice; explain to pt. & family the importance of careful monitoring every 3–6 months by an orthopedic specialist; offer to assist family with further information if it is desired.

2) Psychosocial Adjustment

The child/youth & family will express fears of the unknown and concerns over treatment restrictions; the child/youth & family will express a feeling that they are not alone in facing consequences of diagnosis and treatment; the child/youth will express a belief that s/he has an important part in the successful treatment plan:

— know that both child & family will be anxious about the condition of scoliosis: what it is, how bad it is, how involved the treatment will be; encourage them to air their concerns (embarrassment, peer rejection, abnormal body image for the youth) and fears for the child's well-being, the expense & discomfort of medical visits &

treatment, the guilt over not noticing something abnormal sooner;

— assess the need for knowledge & reassurance, the quality of the relationship between child & family, the obstacles to successful treatment; offer to provide explanations to absent family members or friends whose opinions & attitudes will significantly affect the success of treatment;

— allow time for questions; after consultation with the specialist, reinforce or repeat what was said about the child's condition & recommended plan of treatment; usually the MD will show the x-rays & provide the initial explanation; spend time with the youth while the parents are with the MD; establish trust, explore feelings, & help youth accept responsibility for cooperation with treatment plan.

3) Exercises	The child/youth will accept responsibility for and perform all prescribed exercises twice daily; the child/youth will preserve muscle tone necessary to maintain achieved curvature correction: — know that physical therapist will usually teach & have pt. demonstrate the exercises designed to strengthen abdominal & back muscles & to improve posture; exercises include those of tilting the pelvis so the small of the back is against the floor (supine position) or against the wall (standing), tightening buttock & abdominal muscles, controlled deep-breathing & push-ups with pelvic tilt; observe the pt. doing them at home, school, or clinic; reinforce teaching that each exercise should be done 10–25 times, twice daily, or as prescribed; praise & encourage correct performance of exercises & positive attitudes displayed; — urge & remind child to get in the habit of sitting up straight & standing erect with weight equally distributed on both feet; don't nag, but reinforce the idea that the child only hurts self when s/he uses poor posture or skips exercises.
4) Orthosis (Milwaukee Brace, Boston Brace, or TLSO Jacket)	The patient will accept the responsibility for wearing and caring for the brace or jacket; the patient may express negative feelings but will agree to accept necessary activity restrictions in order to achieve a strong, healthy, straighter back; the patient's family will cooperate with treatment plan and will provide the patient with physical and psychosocial support; the patient will be free of curvature progression, problems of an ill-fitting orthotic device, and psychosocial maladjustment: — introduce the pt. & family to the orthotic device using pictures of other youths wearing them while participating in various sports & recreational activities; provide moral support & encouragement to both parents & youth regarding possible outcomes, but be careful to make no promises about surgery being unnecessary; utilize success stories so that youth can identify with others in similar circumstances;

- know & teach that brace or jacket must be worn 23 hours a day with 30 minutes out morning & evening for exercises and general hygiene; provide the pt. with verbal & written instructions regarding proper application (over a t-shirt but under pants), skin care (keep clean, dry, protect pressure points), brace care (mild soap & water cleansing, saddle soap to leather parts), exercises, restriction of activities (no body-contact sports, weight lifting, horseback riding, gymnastics, trampoline, or driving);
- schedule a team conference (parent, teacher, school nurse, counselor) with pt. & best friend to provide information, explore feelings & attitudes, arrange for PE class activity substitutes, & plan seating & desk top height adjustments PRN;
- have parents arrange for parties, dances, private home sessions with friends, & other suitable activities so child/youth will not withdraw from socializing;
- suggest that parent take youth to orthodontist for assessment of jaw alignment because of pressure from chin rest on brace (not needed for underarm jacket type);
- stress importance of regular, frequent follow-up appointments to ensure proper brace/jacket fit & effective wear; share progress as shown on periodic x-rays.

Discharge Planning and Teaching Objectives/Outcomes:

1) (The Child/Youth and Parents) Verbalize an understanding of scoliosis, the child's condition, treatment aims, and anticipated outcomes of selected therapeutic regimen.
2) Have written instructions regarding exercises, orthotic device care and wear, restrictions of activities, frequency of scoliosis follow-up check-ups. State a willingness to adhere to regimen and demonstrate ability to follow instructions correctly and faithfully.
3) Have suitable plan to meet psychosocial and physical needs of patient.
4) Agree to keep appointments as ordered for continuing medical observation and x-rays to ensure correction is maintained.

Recommended References

"Carol, A Girl With Bracing," by B. Anderson. *American Journal of Nursing*, September 1979:1589–1598.

"The Patient With Scoliosis: The Defect—Classification and Detection; The Orthoplastic Jacket," by C. Holt de Toledo. *American Journal of Nursing*, September 1979:1589–1598.

Scoliosis—A Handbook for Patients. Chicago: Scoliosis Research Society (430 Michigan Ave., 60611).

"Scoliosis Screening: An Approach Used In the School," by D. Miller and C. Lever. *Journal of School Health*, February 1982:98–101.

"Spotting Scoliosis Sooner." *Emergency Medicine*, May 15, 1980:106–108.

"You Can Help Children With Scoliosis." *Patient Care*, April 30, 1981:111–127.

The Child/Youth with Scoliosis: Surgical Management

LONG TERM GOAL: The child/youth will recover from a surgical correction of spinal curvature, free of preventable complications; will accept responsibility for cooperating with a prolonged convalescence and therapeutic regimen; will attain and maintain a structurally balanced spinal column, centered torso, and improved alignment.

General Considerations:

— Read NCPG #4:28, "The Child/Youth with Scoliosis: Medical Management."

— **Surgical treatment** is indicated for severe, rigid curvatures of 40°–70° and especially for double major curves when whole spine is involved. After skeletal traction to stretch muscles and ligaments, spinal fusion is performed in one or two stages. A Risser localizer body cast (of Hexelite, fiberglass, or plaster) is worn postoperatively for three to 12 months, depending on the patient's age and type of scoliosis.

— **Nursing responsibilities** (surgical and orthopedic clinic) **preoperatively** include knowing surgical treatment plan and expected outcomes, assessing physical and psychologic status of the patient, and preparing the patient and family to cope with the stress of surgery.

— **Nursing responsibilities postoperatively** include providing measures to facilitate recovery, to prevent complications, and to ensure successful outcomes of spinal curvature correction; and preparing the patient and family to assume complete care at home in cooperation with orthopedist's therapeutic regimen.

— Refer to the following guides as applicable: NCPGs #2:41–43, "General Post-op Care, Parts A, B, and C;" #2:44, "General Pre-op Care;" #2:45, "Hazards of Immobility;" and #2:50, "Traction: General Principles"

Specific Considerations, Potential Patient Outcomes, and Nursing Actions:

1) Prevention of Complications

The patient will be free of preventable complications (infections, neurologic deficits, skin trauma, immobilization hazards, sensory deprivation):

— refer to NCPG #3:08, "The Patient with a Laminectomy/Spinal Fusion;"

— ascertain that parents & pt. understand the complete course of treatment & possible outcomes; know that pre-op the pt. often has traction to stretch muscles & ligaments, then spinal fusion (anterior or posterior approach) in one or two stages, then a Risser body cast (*sometimes* used alone after traction instead of surgery) to stabilize spine throughout healing period, and, finally, a brace & physiotherapy to regain muscle strength & limb function;

- assist with the application of traction & cast, taking care to calm the child/youth; explain sensations to be expected (loss of sense of balance, discomfort of maintaining position throughout procedure, fear of unknown); refer to NCPGs #2:09, "The Patient with a Cast," and #2:34, "Cast Care: General Principles;"
- after traction or cast is applied, observe & report any signs of neurologic problems (diminished swallow, loss of lateral gaze & ability to follow a moving finger, cranial & spinal cord responses) headache, weakness, pain, incontinence, hyperreflexia of lower extremities, or dysesthesia (impairment of sensitivity, pins & needles sensation) of hands or feet; clearly understand whether you are to remove traction or cut cast immediately if notification of & observation by an MD cannot be quickly accomplished; with prompt recognition & correction, these untoward signs are reversible & permanent neurological injury can be avoided;
- observe for skin redness & irritation caused by diminished circulation & pressure; be certain that stockinette, foam pads, & sheepskin pads are properly placed; keep skin clean, dry, & free of irritants;
- if pt. in "dynamic" type traction, encourage the exercise movements that activate the traction pull; balance exercise with rest periods to avoid undue fatigue;
- if pt. movement is restricted, demonstrate acceptable movements & encourage flexion-extension foot & knee exercises; use foot rest & trochanter rolls;
- if Stryker or Foster frame or CircOlectric bed used, ensure proper instructions & turning by staff & family;
- if pt. in "halo-femoral" skeletal traction, clean skull pin sites with antiseptic solution BID, gently removing crusts & exudates; cover ends of pins for safety; be careful not to jar or bump traction parts;
- monitor & record vital signs, I&O, weight, color, appearance & specific gravity of urine;
- coughing & deep-breathing exercises Q2H;
- know that because a Dwyer-type fusion requires an anterior surgical approach with a thoracotomy, chest tube drainage will be in place; mechanical ventilation may be needed; prepare pt. & family in advance so they will know what to expect; refer to NCPG #1:34, "Chest Tubes and Bottles: Water-seal Drainage;"
- maintain patency & proper operation of CVP line, nasogastric suction, & Foley catheter; record when these are removed & normal function has been re-established; continue to assess bowel & bladder function; give laxatives or suppositories PRN; observe for signs of bladder retention or infection;
- monitor IV administration to ensure adequate urinary output (25–30 m/H) while preventing fluid overload;
- when bowel sounds return, advance pt. from liquids to solid foods (usually a high protein, low calorie diet) as tolerated; force fluids to reduce the likelihood of urinary tract infection;

— supervise range-of-motion exercises QID; refer to NCPG #1:47;
— involve family in the care of the pt. as soon as possible, teaching & showing them effective & safe measures; encourage the pt. to do as much for self as able (to reduce depression, dependency, frustration);
— observe & investigate all pt. complaints promptly (anorexia, nausea, vomiting, pain in chest, shortness of breath, rapid breathing or heartbeat, pain in legs, abdomen, or elsewhere); report to MD promptly; ascertain & correct cause before administering analgesics & sedatives; know that post-op pain, following Harrington procedure, is expected & considerable for 3–4 days; give IM analgesics PRN as ordered;
— when body cast is applied & dry, help pt. deal with realities of limitation; explore feelings of claustrophobia & depression; teach pt. safe methods of movement; if ambulation permitted, assist pt. with first attempts, because of dizziness & balance problems; reassure female adolescents that body cast has no effect on breast development or menstrual periods; tell pt. cast will be changed as body grows; review NCPG #2:29, "The Patient Experiencing a Body Image Disturbance;"
— provide pt. with radio, TV, social interaction with staff & other pts.; encourage visitors; provide prism glasses for reading; place items within reach.

2) Patient/Family Education — The parent (or care giver) will express knowledge and confidence in caring for the patient at home; the parent will successfully prevent complications necessitating rehospitalization:
— review NCPG #3:32, "Teaching the Parent/Guardian/Child: General Suggestions;"
— discharge plans include:
  - suggestions for rental of hospital bed or safe elevation of standard bed
  - use of bedboard, firm mattress, foot board, trapeze or rope pull-up
  - desirable equipment: fracture bedpan, bed tray, prism glasses for reading or watching TV, pedestal mirror, absorbent pads or disposable diapers (for use when giving mouth care, using bedpan, shampooing hair)
  - feeding & diet instructions (aimed at providing fibrous bulk & preventing weight gain)
  - skin care & prevention of pressure sores
  - positioning, turning, deep breathing, & exercises; elimination aids
  - fire safety precautions & emergency evacuation procedures
  - tips for diversion & morale; time off for the care giver;
— encourage the parent to express doubts, fears, worry over doing what is needed for child; urge contact with home health nurse for any problems that parent can't solve satisfactorily; tell family members that pt.'s feel-

ings of anger, depression, apathy, & dependence are normal & expected; help them to look at ways they can respond & cope to reduce family tensions & to improve family relationships;

— arrange for tutoring, classes by telephone & TV, periodic visits from school district's home teacher; provide earphones for use of radio, TV, & tape recorder;

— if possible, arrange to meet a family who has had similar situations & successfully managed;

— when the pt. is permitted up, s/he should resume as much self-care & as many normal activities as possible; encourage the child/youth to assume responsibility for daily exercises & physical therapy.

Discharge Planning and Teaching Objectives/Outcomes:

1) (Child/Family) Has specific written instructions from orthopedic surgeon regarding permitted activities, diet, exercises, care of cast, and date of return medical appointment.
2) Has demonstrated competence and cooperation with home care plan developed by nurse and family.
3) Can plan meals from a nutritionally balanced diet that will meet age/activity needs without excessive weight gain.
4) Has name, phone number of referrals for assistance with home care, physical therapy, education, and mental health counseling.
5) Has stated intention to keep regular appointments with doctor/clinic at recommended three to six month intervals through lengthy treatment and rehabilitation period.
6) Knows to tell OB/GYN doctor about scoliosis correction when pregnant (5°–8° shifts in curvature can occur during this period).

Recommended References

"By Losing Control of Herself, Linda Controlled Her Parents . . . and Us," by B. Faro. *Nursing 80*, April 1980:62–64.

"Cast Care: General Principles." *NCP Guide #2:34*, 2nd Ed., Nurseco, 1980.

"Chest Tubes and Bottles: Water-seal Drainage." *NCP Guide #1:34*, 2nd Ed., Nurseco, 1980.

"The Child/Youth with Scoliosis: Medical Management." *NCP Guide #4:28*, 2nd Ed., Nurseco, 1983.

"General Postoperative Care, Parts A, B, and C." *NCP Guides #2:41–43*, 2nd Ed., Nurseco, 1980.

"General Pre-op Care." *NCP Guide #2:44*, 2nd Ed., Nurseco, 1980.

"Hazards of Immobility." *NCP Guide #2:45*, 2nd Ed., Nurseco, 1980.

"The Patient Experiencing a Body Image Disturbance." *NCP Guide #2:29*, 2nd Ed., Nurseco, 1980.

"The Patient with a Cast." *NCP Guide #2:09*, 2nd Ed., Nurseco, 1980.

"The Patient with a Laminectomy/Spinal Fusion." *NCP Guide #3:08*, 2nd Ed., Nurseco, 1983.

"The Patient With Scoliosis—Surgical Management and Nursing Care," by L. Micheli et al., and "Spinal Fusion: Emotional Stress and Adjustment," by L. Schatzinger, et al. *American Journal of Nursing*, September 1979:1599–1612.

"Range of Motion Exercises." *NCP Guide #1:47*, 2nd Ed., Nurseco, 1980.

"Teaching the Parent/Guardian/Child: General Suggestions." *NCP Guide #3:32*, 2nd Ed., Nurseco, 1983.

"Traction: General Principles." *NCP Guide #2:50*, 2nd Ed., Nurseco, 1981.

The Mother who Breast-Feeds Her Infant

LONG TERM GOAL: The mother will express satisfaction with breast-feeding and experience feelings of closeness and bonding with infant.

General Considerations:

— **Benefits of breast-feeding** include:
- human milk is more readily assimilated than cow's milk
- increased immunological protection for infant, fewer allergies, less tendency for obesity, less colic
- colostrum, the forerunner of milk, is nutritious and provides antibody protection
- early suckling at the breast assists mother in promoting normal involution of uterus and thus preventing postpartum hemorrhage
- provision of a unique emotional bond between mother and infant that forms the basis of a close, enduring relationship
- the incidence of breast cancer is reported to be lower in women who have breast-fed.

— **Physiology of breast-feeding:** *antepartally*, estrogen stimulates breast growth and prepares breasts for lactation by promoting growth of ducts. Progesterone matures milk glands (lobules) and stimulates acini cells. Secretion of milk from the mother's breast is most often initiated when the baby suckles. Suckling stimulates the nipple, sending nerve impulses travelling from the nipple to the *posterior pituitary*, which stimulates *oxytocin*. Oxytocin stimulates *prolactin* (released from the anterior pituitary) and, in the breast, it stimulates the muscles surrounding the milk glands. These muscles contract and force the milk to be expelled and received by the infant (let-down reflex). Prolactin stimulates milk secretion. Oxytocin works specifically on myoepithelial cells. Milk production is on an on-demand basis; therefore, an increase in breast stimulation (i.e., frequent feedings) will increase milk production.

— **The engorgement period** occurs around second or third postpartal day. Electric hand pumps or manual expression may be used. If infant is in NICU, breast milk may be stored in bottles and refrigerated for later feeding. Excess breast milk may be used in breast milk banks; techniques and storage standards vary.

— Breast-feeding is not a reliable form of birth control, although it is known to reduce the incidence of pregnancy.

— **Nursing responsibilities** include helping to make breast-feeding a pleasurable and effective experience for mother and infant, assessing mother's level of knowledge in area of breast care and nutrition, and health teaching as necessary.

Specific Considerations, Potential Patient Outcomes, and Nursing Actions:

1) Education of Mother and Infant

The mother will experience success and satisfaction with breast-feeding; the mother will assist her infant to suckle/"latch on:"

— before initial feeding experience (if possible), assess what the mother knows & feels about breast-feeding; many new mothers feel they will not have enough milk or that they will be working soon & therefore can't breast-feed successfully (not true); assure her that she will be able to produce enough milk & that the baby will be able to feed properly, pointing out that the infant, as well as the mother, may have to go through an initial learning period;

— share with mother that if she plans to return to work in 6–8 weeks & wishes to continue nursing, she has several alternatives: (a) hand expression of breast milk; (b) breast-pump expression; (c) formula supplementation of milk production of breasts (only if necessary); or (d) have baby brought to her or return home on break.

— initiate breast-feeding as soon after birth as possible for all mothers, including cesarean-section mothers, since it helps nurture bonding; be aware that healthy babies do their best suckling in the first 2 hours after birth;

— to help baby to the breast, demonstrate rooting reflex by gently patting area around baby's mouth so that mouth will open; be sure that baby latches on to the areola & not just the nipple (this could make nipples bleed); if necessary, wake baby up before & during feeding in order to promote the feeding process;

— teach mother to position baby properly so baby won't have to turn its head to feed & can look up at mother while feeding ("en face" position);

— arrange for demand feedings in order to satisfy infant & decrease breast engorgement;

— explain to the mother that the let-down reflex is affected by anxiety, fear, etc., & discuss ways she can relax (e.g., 15 minutes before feeding time, place warm compresses on breasts, play soothing music, etc.); listen to mother's feelings & concerns about breast-feeding, parenting, resuming role as wife/lover/worker;

— if immediate weaning is necessary, explore & be sensitive to mother's feelings & offer emotional support;

— know that nipple aids can help with breast-feeding, but are not always successful;

— give mother information re: support groups for breast-feeding mothers: La Leche League (local chapters); CARESS, a C-section group supportive of mothers who are breast-feeding & have had a cesarean section; breast-feeding infant clinics (at various medical centers);

— provide printed materials on breast-feeding.

2) Care of Breasts

The mother will care for her breasts daily in order to avoid infection and to ensure comfort during the lactation period; the mother will remain free of sore or cracked nipples:

— ensure that mother wears a nursing bra to provide support & comfort;
— teach mother to wash hands well before breast-feeding & to cleanse breasts gently before & after each feeding, using only warm water on breasts, no soaps;
— apply nipple cream, such as pure lanolin, in order to keep nipples soft & pliable & to prevent cracks that may predispose her to hard, inflamed nipples & increase susceptibility to infection/mastitis;
— teach woman to leave nipples open to air when possible so as to decrease friction of tight bra, especially with breast pads, & to keep free of moisture from leakage (moisture could be a breeding place for bacteria); change breast pads frequently;
— provide Woolwich breast shields to help inverted nipples; demonstrate nipple-rolling exercises to toughen up normal or flat nipples (can be helpful even if not begun prenatally);
— tell mother that daily care of nipples is the best method to prevent sore or cracked nipples.

3) Prevention of Complications

The mother will remain free of preventable problems and complications, e.g., engorgement, mastitis:

— assess mother's ability to carry out proper method of manual expression of milk; health teach PRN;
— for the cesarean-section mother who is breast-feeding, help with positions that will avoid discomfort, i.e., lateral Sims' position, football hold for feeding, etc.;
— ensure that mother knows correct positioning of fingers around areola (fingers underneath areola & thumb above, being sure to keep fingers away from the areola);
— relieve discomfort of engorgement by applying warm, moist compresses &/or express milk by hand/pump;
— monitor mother for early signs/symptoms of mastitis/infection (fever; chills; general malaise; breast tenderness; reddened, indurated area surrounding breast; painful breast); should any appear, provide warm compresses to area, get an order for acetaminophen PRN (do not stop nursing); if signs & symptoms of infection increase or abscess appears, check with MD re antibiotics & manually express milk until infection clears; infant may feed on unaffected side until mastitis clears;
— know that routine nipple shields, except for fully inverted nipples, are not always helpful; most times, the infant will be able to help stimulate the nipple to erection;
— know that breast-milk jaundice is often only a transient problem; breast-feeding is interrupted for approximately 48 hours & then resumed.

4) Nutrition — The mother will ingest a diet sufficient to provide adequate nutrition for self and infant:
- teach mother to eat a diet similar to that of pregnancy with slight increase in overall caloric intake;
- discuss drugs & foods that pass through breast milk (all drugs do; some foods may cause diarrhea, constipation, allergies in infant [will vary among individuals]) and effects of smoking & alcohol on breast milk;
- be aware that women on birth-control pills should not be breast-feeding (pills decrease milk production; estrogens/progestins are passed on to infant via breast milk & their effect on infant is unknown);
- discuss the importance of increased fluid intake while nursing (should be approximately 2–3 glasses over normal daily intake);
- assure mother that there is no need for supplemental feedings for baby, especially at initiation of breast-feeding; they can inhibit firm establishment of breast-feeding; many breast-fed babies go from breast milk to solids at about 5–6 months of age.

Discharge Planning and Teaching Objectives/Outcomes

1) (The Mother) Knows baby's need to nurse more frequently in the early weeks, sometimes eight to 12 times per day.
2) Puts baby's needs first; has someone to help her with chores at home while she attends to infant's needs.
3) Knows that she will experience an increased need for rest and has made realistic provisions for this.
4) Has telephone number of doctor, nurse practitioner, or support organizations for counseling for problems.
5) Has diet instructions. Understands care of her breasts. Has instructions regarding weaning; knows it is slow and gradual.

Recommended References

"Basics for Breastfeeding," by J. Riordan and B. Countryman. *JOGN Nursing*, Parts 1 & 2, July/August 1980:207–213; Parts 3 & 4, September/October 1980:273–283; Parts 5 & 6, November/December 1980:357–366.

"Breastfeeding and the Working Mother," by M. Broome. *JOGN Nursing*, May/June 1981:201–202.

"Breastfeeding Works for Caesareans, Too," by K. Frantz and B. Kalman. *RN*, December 1979:38–47.

"Drugs for Two in Lactation," by S. Wicklund. *American Journal of Nursing*, September 1982:1428–1430.

"Important Factors in Breastfeeding Success," by E. Beske and M. Gawes. *MCN: The American Journal of Maternal Child Nursing*, May/June 1982:174–179.

"Improving Nipple Graspability for Success at Breastfeeding," by K. Cadwell. *JOGN Nursing*, July/August 1981:277–279.

"A Key to Successful Breastfeeding in a Non-Supportive Culture, " by H. Meara. *Journal of Nurse-Midwifery*, Spring 1976: 20–26.

Nutrition in Pregnancy and Lactation, by S. Williams. St. Louis: Mosby, 1977.

"Possible Related Risks to Breastfeeding," by R. Serie. *JOGN Nursing*, January/February 1982:34–36.

"Selecting the Right Breast Pump," by E. Tibbets and K. Cadwell. *MCN: The American Journal of Maternal Child Nursing*, July/August 1980:262–264.

You Can Breastfeed Your Baby...Even in Special Situations, by D. Brewster. Emmaus, PA: Rodale Press, 1979.

The Mother with a Cesarean Birth

LONG TERM GOAL: The mother will experience her hospital stay as a "birthing experience" rather than as an operative procedure; the mother will have optimal recovery from surgery.

General Considerations:

— **Types of cesarean births:** primary and repeat. Trends point to an increased number of vaginal births following a previous cesarean, especially for women whose previous section was for fetal distress or breech presentation. The indication for the prior C-section is a strong determinant in whether or not vaginal birth is an option.

— **Indications** for cesarean birth fall into two categories: *maternal* and/or *fetal*. Maternal reasons include cephalopelvic disproportion, failure to progress in labor, diabetes, and other medical/obstetrical complications. Fetal reasons include fetal distress and abnormal presentation.

— **Incidence** has increased over the last few years, with rates as high as 20%–30% in some communities. Possible reasons for this are an increased number of older primiparas, increased tendency to section for breech presentation, the desire to attain safer fetal outcomes, inappropriate response to fetal monitoring data, and medico-legal implications affecting fetal morbidity/perinatal outcomes.

— **Tests for fetal lung maturity** are usually done prior to elective cesarean section, i.e., amniocentesis for L/S ratio and other enzymatic tests (now in research) that assess lung maturity in the infant to avoid iatrogenic prematurity.

— **Types of incisions:** classical, low classical, and low traverse with possible Pfannenstiel skin incision (bikini-cut incision).

— **Nursing responsibilities** include caring for the mother as both a postoperative and a postpartum patient, providing pre- and postoperative teaching, monitoring the patient's physical status postoperatively for early signs of complications, and aiding parent-infant bonding.

Specific Considerations, Potential Patient Outcomes, and Nursing Actions:

1) Pre-op Care — The mother will experience only a moderate amount of anxiety for self and baby; the mother will know what to expect postoperatively in terms of ambulation, discomfort, contact with baby;

— assess level of anxiety, understanding, & feelings; discuss with mother/father/significant other (SO) reason(s) for C-section; provide as much information as she wants & needs; know that doing too much pre-op teaching without assessing how much she wants to know can lead to increased anxiety;

— if emergency C-section, be aware that pt. may be overwhelmed with all that is happening; take time to allow pt. to express her feelings & to explain procedures & rationale (this will give a measure of comfort & reassurance); try to provide as much information to mother/couple as possible, especially since she may have general anesthesia for a "crash C-section;"
— provide information regarding what to expect postpartally in terms of discomfort, ambulation, infant contact, positioning, anesthesia options; explain pre-op procedures (Foley, prep, anesthesia); refer to NCPG #2:44, "General Pre-op Care;"
— obtain operative permits & baseline data on vital signs;
— arrange with nurses in OR/delivery room for parents to have some contact with infant at birth; if possible, keep couples together in section room (if parents had planned to be together in delivery room, they can be very upset at the prospect of being separated for a cesarean).

2) Post-op/ Postpartum Care

The parent(s) will express pleasure in accomplishment of successful delivery of their child; the mother will be free of preventable postoperative complications:
— ask if there was parent-infant contact in OR; if not, arrange for this in recovery room;
— monitor vital signs, urinary output, pain level; observe for signs of shock; check amount & character of lochia; check incision; "gas pains" & "pain" are often common complaints; refer to NCPGs #2:41-43, "General Post-op Care;"
— arrange for initial breast-feeding (if mother plans to nurse infant) as soon after C-section birth as possible (early breast-feeding helps promote bonding); refer to NCPG #4:30, "The Mother Who Breast-Feeds her Infant;"
— assess for responses, feelings, & concerns about C-section birth; give emotional support by accepting feelings & by active listening;
— health teach mother re positioning techniques (especially to help the breast-feeding mother) & relaxation techniques;
— check with MD re having mother start post-op exercises, such as abdominal-tightening exercise to reduce gas discomfort; go over exercises with mother to ensure she understands them; refer to NCPG #3:31, "Postpartum Exercises;"
— assess mothering-role capabilities & do patient teaching as needed; refer to NCPG #3:28, "The Normal Postpartum Patient;"

- be aware that a major concern of these mothers is feelings of inadequacy in caring for their babies; to alleviate this, ensure that the mother has all supplies she needs for baby close at hand, help her find positions of comfort while feeing baby, rearrange IV tubing PRN, etc.;
- know that early discharge (usually 5 days) for these mothers is now current practice.

3) Parent-Infant Bonding — The parent(s) will display behaviors indicating initial bonding to infant:

- refer to NCPG #4:32, "Parent-Infant Bonding;"
- assist with bonding techniques (eye contact, touch, etc.) as early as possible;
- if mother is unable to have physical contact, arrange for father or other family members to begin attachment process with infant;
- if infant has complications & must be separated, accompany mother or couple to nursery, keep news of infant up-to-date for family as much as possible; arrange for person caring for baby to speak with couple regarding infant's condition;
- support liberal visiting policy for father/family;
- know that during surgery there is sensory overload & a stressful physical environment with altered perceptions of the body, heightened fears for self & baby (the latter varies, depending on type of anesthesia); know that providing human contact & early bonding with infant allays many fantasies/fears;
- be aware that mothers who undergo a surgical procedure at time of birth & who are deprived of contact with infant often focus on themselves & their own body rather than on the baby; early bonding with infant can change this, thereby normalizing the process of role change.

Discharge Planning and Teaching Objectives/Outcomes

1) (The mother) Has a referral to a visiting nurse service and/or clinic/doctor appointment for follow-up care.
2) Has telephone numbers to call for counseling and/or emergencies.
3) Has instructions regarding exercises, breast care, breast-feeding, diet, medication, and contraception.
4) Verbalizes confidence in ability to care for infant and in mothering role. Home environment is suitable for infant. Has appropriate help at home.
5) Knows of support groups that are available to cesarean section couples/women: e.g., CARESS, C-SEC, among other community groups/associations.

Recommended References

"Breastfeeding Works for Caesareans, Too," by K. Frantz and B. Kalman. *RN*, December 1979:38–47.
"Cesarean Birth," by J. Stichler and D. Alfonso. *American Journal of Nursing*, March 1980:466-468.
"Cesarean Birth: A Real Family Affair," by K. Hedahl. *American Journal of Nursing*, March 1980:471–472.
The Caesarean Birth Experience, by B. Donovan. Boston: Beacon Press, 1977 (paperback).
The Cesarean Experience: Theoretical and Clinical Perspectives, by C. Kehoe, Ed. New York: Appleton-Century-Crofts, 1981.
"Comparison of Primiparas' Perceptions of Vaginal and Cesarean Births," by J. Marut and R. Mercer. *Nursing Research*, September/October 1979:260–266.
Essential Exercises for the Childbearing Years, by E. Noble (special exercises for C-section patients). Boston: Houghton, Mifflin, 1976.
"The Family-Centered Cesarean Delivery," by S. Bayel and P. Mahon. *MCN: The American Journal of Maternal Child Nursing*, May/June 1980:176–180.
"General Postoperative Care, Parts, A, B, and C." *NCP Guides #2:41-43*, 2nd Ed., Nurseco, 1980.
"General Preoperative Care." *NCP Guide #2:44*, 2nd Ed., Nurseco, 1980.
"The Mother who Breast-Feeds Her Infant." *NCP Guide #4:30*, 2nd Ed., Nurseco, 1983.
"Needs of Cesarean Birth Parents," by J. Fawcett. *JOGN Nursing*, September/October 1981:372.
"The Normal Postpartum Patient." *NCP Guide #3:38*, 2nd Ed., Nurseco, 1983.
"Parent-Infant Bonding." *NCP Guide #4:32*, 2nd Ed., Nurseco, 1983.
"Postpartum Exercises." *NCP Guide #3:31*, 2nd Ed., Nurseco, 1983,
"The Special Needs of the Cesarean Mother," by J Marut. *MCN: The American Journal of Maternal Child Nursing*, July/August 1978:202–206.
"Women's Reactions," by J. Stickler and D. Alfonso. *American Journal of Nursing*, March 1980:468–470.

Parent-Infant Bonding

Definition: Bonding (or attachment) is a unique relationship between two people that is specific and endures through time. It incorporates components of the acquaintance process (i.e., touch, eye-to-eye contact). The acquaintance process is the foundation of subsequent human relationships and is an opportunity for a two-way interaction between responding individuals.

LONG TERM GOAL: The parent(s) and infant will perform attachment behaviors during the critical perinatal period to help ensure the beginning of a good relationship.

General Considerations:

— **Antepartally**, the promotion of bonding begins. A woman "binds in" or attaches herself to the idea of being pregnant and then later, as infant becomes more real and fetal movement is felt, she attaches herself to infant with nesting activities, proper eating habits, "making a good baby," buying clothes that enhance her physical attractiveness, and by gaining weight. She takes pleasure inwardly and exhibits outward expressions of her attachment to her fetus.

— **During the intrapartum period**, a woman must begin to recognize and cue into child's behavior; the infant must do the same (reciprocal interaction). Some of these behavioral cues are orienting behaviors (eye-to-eye contact), active physical-contact behaviors (embracing, clinging, grasping), and signaling behaviors (crying, smiling, vocalizing).

— **Postpartum**, interactive variables affecting bonding include:

a) *in the mother*: touch; eye-to-eye contact; high-pitched voice; entrainment (parents must receive some response signal such as eye movements to begin to form a close bond); time-correlation (mother and infant adjust to other's body rhythms); passive immunity; nasal flora, odor, and heat.

b) *in the infant*: eye-to-contact, crying, oxytocin stimulation, prolactin stimulation, odor, and entrainment. Maternal and infant behaviors complement each other in several sensory and motor systems, thus increasing the probability of interaction.

— **Bonding experiences** need to be promoted for both parents as early as possible. Indicators that bonding is occurring are: fondling, kissing, cuddling, prolonged gazing. These behaviors serve to maintain contact between parent(s) and child and allow expression of affection.

— **Nursing responsibilities** include assessing bonding behaviors and manipulating variables that will increase the degree of bonding.

Specific Considerations, Potential Patient Outcomes, and Nursing Actions:

1) Promotion of Bonding

The parent(s) will display behaviors indicating attachment to their infant:

— know that the first few hours & days after birth are crucial for parent-infant bonding;
— in birthing room, promote placing infant skin-to-skin on mother's undraped abdomen immediately after birth; encourage mother to reach down & touch baby; try to delay silver nitrate application until after mother has had time to hold & fondle infant;
— arrange for father to participate in birth process (i.e., cutting umbilical cord, skin-to-skin contact, help hold/touch infant), to interact with infant (bathe & dress infant), & to help in feeding process if applicable (men often need to be encouraged to do this);
— after birth, arrange for privacy so that parent(s) & child can have extended periods of time to get to know infant & for infant to begin to know them;
— consider sibling bonding; now that many siblings are able to view births, their bonding experiences with infant need to be considered/explored;
— with a *premature infant* or infant that is separated from mother for any reason, telephone contact, eye-to-eye contact, touching, & special visiting privileges help to promote bonding (separation is often a time in which attachment activities are delayed);
— be aware that in bonding with *twins*, parents become optimally attached to only 1 infant at a time; a mother/parent(s) with twins must work with each child individually in the getting-acquainted process;
— with babies with severe *congenital malformations* or infants being *relinquished* for *adoption*, to promote bonding can be cruel; however, the parent(s) should have the opportunity & the reality of holding & inspecting infant; in order to separate (even gradually), one must bond or attach in some way;
— be alert to any indications that may suggest potential neglect or abuse.

2) Parent Education

The parent(s) will state at least five factors that affect the bonding process; the parents know what to expect in terms of growth and development of their infant for the next month:

— at least 1 day before discharge, assess bonding behaviors of parents & child; discuss with parents & health teach PRN;
— assess parent(s)'s knowledge of growth & development of their infant; teach them to be aware of infant's cues, point out baby's strengths as potential individual; refer to NCPGs #3:22, 23, "Normal Growth & Development, Newborn, Infant;"

— discuss parent-infant bonding as a gradual process occurring over time; explain the role of reciprocal interaction & point out specific interactive behaviors;
— refer to Brazelton's Neonatal Behavioral Assessment Scale to help parents identify each baby's unique qualities.

Discharge Planning and Teaching Objectives/Outcomes:

1) (The Parent(s)) Has/have an awareness of the attachment process and can state where s/he feels s/he is in the process.
2) Knows that bonding to a premature infant or to an infant with congenital abnormalities takes time.
3) Has made appointments for follow-up telephone contact, home visit, to promote the process.
4) Has a referral to a VNA, clinic, or doctor's office to work specifically on attachment (for those parents who are having a problem identifying or attaching to infant).

Recommended References

"Anxiety as a Potential Factor Affecting Maternal Attachment," by K. Avant. *JOGN Nursing*, November/December 1981:416–419.
"Assessing Maternal Attachment: First Step Toward the Prevention of Child Abuse," by J. Hurd. *JOGN Nursing*, July/August 1975:25–30.
"Binding-In in the Postpartum Period," by R. Rubin. *MCN: The American Journal of Maternal Child Nursing*, Summer 1977:67–75.
"A Conceptual Framework of Bonding," by J. Gay. *JOGN Nursing*, November/December 1981:440–444.
"Early Postpartum Separation and Maternal Attachment to Twins," by P. Dickerson. *JOGN Nursing*, March/April 1981:120–123.
"Engrossment: the Newborn's Impact upon the Father," by M. Greenberg and N. Morris. *The American Journal of Orthopsychiatry*, July 1974:520–531.
"Making Baby's Acquaintance," by P. Geary et al. *MCN: The American Journal of Maternal Child Nursing*, January/February 1982:37–41.
"Maternal-Infant Attachment in a Traditional Hospital Setting," by S. Paukert. *JOGN Nursing*, January/February 1982:23–26.
"Maternal, Paternal and Infant Interaction in the Early Postpartum Period," by D. Chally. Kansas City, MO: American Nurses' Association, Division on Maternal and Child Health Nursing Practice, 1979.
Neonatal Behavioral Assessment Scale, by T. Brazelton. Philadelphia: Lippincott, 1973.
"Normal Growth and Development: Newborn, Infant." *NCP Guides #3:22, 23*, 2nd Ed., Nurseco, 1983.
"The Nurse's Role in Parent-Infant Bonding—Overview, Assessment, Intervention," by R. Jenkins et al. *JOGN Nursing*, March/April 1981:114–118.
Parent-Infant Bonding, by M. Klaus and J. Kennell, 2nd Ed. St. Louis: Mosby, 1982.
"Paternal-Infant Bonding in the First-time Father," by A. Taubenheim. *JOGN Nursing*, July/August 1981:261-264.

The Pregnant Teen

LONG TERM GOAL: The pregnant teen will receive quality care, counseling, and referral services to assist her in her mothering role.

General Considerations:

— **Incidence:** teenage pregnancy has increased in recent years. In 1979, one of every six babies born in the US was to a teenage mother.

— Pregnancy causes disruptions in the life cycle of the adolescent, affecting body image and identity formation, specifically female identity; body-image development is not well integrated during adolescence and changes or disruptions in body integrity are often heightened for teens, especially during labor and birth. Read NCPG #2:29, "The Patient Experiencing a Body Image Disturbance." Schooling is also affected; there is either a complete disruption and change of school and friends or the teen is transferred to a special school for pregnant girls.

— **An at-risk obstetrical population** is represented by this group. *Antepartal complications* often include anemia, pre-eclampsia, size-date discrepancy, poor weight gain, and urinary tract infections. During *labor and birth*, *complications* include varying degrees of pre-eclampsia, cephalopelvic disproportion, uterine dysfunction, anemia, and occasional prematurity. Special "teen pregnancy" clinics are available in many cities for teens and their infants.

— **Early-aged pregnant teens** often have limited resources, both financial and social; older adolescents tend to have a stronger supportive network and personal autonomy. Parental and peer pressure and/or support are significant factors.

— **Nursing responsibilities** include counseling to make adolescent aware of options available to her (abortion, adoption, or keeping infant), supporting her choice, assuming the role of patient advocate, helping client integrate body-image changes, assessing and providing for physical needs, and referring to community resources as appropriate. Read NCPG #3:28, "The Normal Postpartum Patient."

Specific Considerations, Potential Patient Outcomes, and Nursing Actions:

1) Psychosocial Adjustment (Antepartum)

The adolescent will discuss her feelings about becoming a mother (or giving up her baby), the client will discuss her future plans for child care and return to school:

— be aware that the provision of antepartum care for the adolescent involves a comprehensive consideration of all types of physical caring & support services;

— sit & talk with teenager away from parents/family; encourage her to discuss what she feels about the changes occurring in her life due to pregnancy ("What is it like for you just now?"); assure her that her feelings are usual & expected, & that others in same situation have similar feelings; allow her to express concerns & fears about giving birth; know that often there is a great deal of fear, resentment (why me?), anxiety, confusion, doubt, & worry about partner's, peers', & parental reactions;
— assess availability & strengths of her support systems, e.g., husband, partner, family, peers; if possible, arrange for a social service consult to evaluate social & family situation (if client chooses adoption or abortion, social service must be contacted):
— if she is undecided whether to keep child, give it up, or have an abortion, help client make decision by providing information, sharing feelings, having her make out a list of the pros & cons of each option, but *do not* make decision for her; refer her to community counseling services PRN;
— discuss plans to return to school (special school programs for the pregnant teen often include pregnancy content in the curriculum) & help the teenager to complete as much schooling as possible;
— know that the initial pelvic exam for the teenage mother can be frightening & psychologically traumatic; attempt to health teach client re knowledge of sexual organs, introduction to the pelvic/speculum exam; using visual aids in the process assists in calming fears & displacing fantasies;
— during labor & birth, nurses often assume the position of patient advocate for teenagers;
— assess knowledge & health teach in small segments, observing her for anxiety; encourage questions.

2) Psychosocial Adjustment (Postpartum)

The adolescent will adapt to the reality of caring for an infant; the teenage mother will initiate bonding with her infant:
— be cognizant of Mercer's (1979) stages of role attainment for the teenage mother:
a) *fairyland phase*: initial attention of gifts & giving that the teen receives after birth adds a sense of unreality to the period after birth;
b) *reality-shock phase*: this period begins shortly after the initial hospital or birthing experience; it reaches a peak the 2nd week postpartum; all the attention & gift-giving initially experienced is overshadowed by the demands of the mothering role; infant becomes more of a reality & more demanding;
c) *give and take phase*: occurs near the 3rd month postpartum; the balance between giving attention & the demands of mothering can come into conflict;

d) *internalization phase*: occurs from the 6th–8th month postpartum; pleasure & gratification in new role are evident;

— know that teen mothers who experience no untoward difficulties with the mothering role are noted to have the following characteristics: supportive mate, a mother who recognizes them as capable of mothering, rewards in mothering role, & family members who help them with infant care;

— review NCPG #4:32, "Parent-Infant Bonding;"

— refer to NCPG #3:28, "The Normal Postpartum Patient," for additional nursing actions.

3) Patient/Family Education — The teen will describe in own words her understanding and knowledge of child care, birth control, and nutrition; the teen mother will begin to adopt the mothering role in gradual phases, incorporating changing beliefs, attitudes, feelings, and self-image:

— teach parent(s) that critical periods for follow-up with infant include: 1st day after birth, 1 month, 3–4 months, 6–9 months, & the importance of keeping these appts.; refer to NCPGs #3:22, 23, "Normal Growth & Development: Infant, Newborn;"

— be aware of the postpartum impact for the teen father; during this time, fathering & decision-making skills regarding infant support are developed;

— provide contraceptive information at a level parent(s) can understand & put to practical use; birth control pills & IUDs are most common methods for females; use of condoms by the teen male will help to decrease the teen birth rate; known that often the contraceptive problem is one of client failure, not method failure; read NCPGs #5:38, 39, "Birth Control Methods;"

— if mother is going to keep her baby, assess basic mothering skills & teach care of baby PRN; encourage rooming-in & extended contact with infant following delivery;

— assess client's dietary habits & health teach PRN; explain food groups & rationale for ingesting an adequate diet; have client select an adequate diet for self & critique it for her.

Discharge Planning and Teaching Objectives/Outcomes

1) (The Client) Has referral to visiting nurse service and/or clinic for follow-up care for self and baby. Has emergency telephone numbers of hospital/clinic/doctor/nurse.
2) Demonstrates an understanding of and verbalizes a plan to use family-planning methods and community services.

3) Has realistic plans to continue schooling.
4) Has a support network available to help her cope with stresses of her new situation/role. Knows community resource groups for teen mothers, such as:
   - March of Dimes
   - Alan Guttmacher Institute, Planned Parenthood of America
   - Child Welfare League of America
   - National Organization on Adolescent Pregnancy and Parenting
   - Department of Health and Human Services, Office of Adolescent Pregnancy Programs, Washington, DC
   - Right to Life, Pro Life

Recommended References

"Adolescent Pregnancies and Problems," by H. Burst. *Journal of Nurse-Midwifery*, March/April 1979:19–24.
"Adolescent Pregnancy," by M. Chanis et al. *Journal of Nurse-Midwifery*, May/June 1979:18–22.
"Birth Control: Permanent, Temporary Methods." *NCP Guides #5:38, 39*, Nurseco, 1981.
"The Children of Teenage Parents," by W. Baldwin and V. Cain. *Family Planning Perspectives*, January/February 1980:34–39.
'A Clinic for Pregnant Teens," by M. Daniels and D. Manning. *American Journal of Nursing*, January 1983:68–71.
"Contraception and Adolescent Pregnancy," by C. Burbach. *JOGN Nursing*, September/October 1980:319–323.
"Counseling the Pregnant Teenager," by J. Admire and L. Byers. *Nursing 81*, April 1981:62–63.
"Normal Growth and Development: Newborn, Infant." *NCP Guides #3:22, 23*, 2nd Ed., Nurseco, 1983.
"The Normal Postpartum Patient." *NCP Guide #3:28*, 2nd Ed., Nurseco, 1983.
"Parent-Infant Bonding." *NCP Guide #4:32*, 2nd Ed., Nurseco, 1983.
"The Patient Experiencing a Body Image Disturbance." *NCP Guide #2:29*, 2nd Ed., Nurseco, 1980.
Perspectives on Adolescent Health Care, by R. Mercer. Philadelphia: Lippincott, 1979.
"Reaching and Helping the Adolescent Who becomes Pregnant," by M. Steinman. *MCN: The American Journal of Maternal Child Nursing*, January/February 1979:35–37.
"A Systems Approach to Adolescent Pregnancy," by S. Panzarine et al. *JOGN Nursing*, 1981:287–289.
"Teenage Motherhood: the First Year. Part 1: The Teenage Mother's Views and Responses. Part 2: How the Infants Fared," by R. Mercer. *JOGN Nursing*, January/February 1980:16–27
Teenage Pregnancy: the Problem that Hasn't Gone Away. New York: Guttmacher Institute, 1981.

The Aged Patient: Chronic Organic Brain Syndrome

Definition: Organic brain syndrome (OBS), also known as organic mental disorder, confusional state, brain failure, senile dementia, or senility, is a mental dysfunction due to the response of the aging brain to disease or damage.

LONG TERM GOAL: The patient will be maintained for as long as possible in a state of bio/psycho/social integrity with as much independence and contact with reality as possible.

General Considerations:

— **Incidence:** affects more than one million Americans.

— **Causes:** *acute* organic brain syndrome may be caused by a wide range of conditions (cardiovascular disease, respiratory disease, metabolic disorders, infection, drug intoxication, dehydration, and electrolyte imbalance); *chronic* organic brain syndrome is caused by Alzheimer's disease (see NCPG #5:02) or cerebrovascular disease (a multi-infarct dementia, formerly called cerebral arteriosclerotic disease).

— **Signs and symptoms:** impaired memory for recent events, disorientation, poor judgment, emotional lability, regressed behavior, altered ability to comprehend accurately, altered ability to cope with fears, fantasies, paranoid delusions or other strange ideas, and confusion.

— **Confusion** is a state of mental disorder, derangement, and perplexion in which attention, comprehension, memory, and perceptions are disturbed or adversely affected. It may be temporary or permanent. It is classified as *functional* or *organic*. Functional confusion has psychosocial or developmental causes and is associated with mental illness. Organic confusion has physical causes (mentioned above) and is termed chronic when applied to the aged person with Alzheimer's or cerebrovascular disease.

— **Treatment** is aimed at correcting the underlying disorder(s), but only 10%–15% of OBS cases are potentially reversible. A therapeutic milieu involving all aspects of good patient management is thought to be beneficial, supportive, and humane for the confused elderly patient.

— **Nursing responsibilities** include planning, intervening, and evaluating to maintain the highest level of bio/psycho/social functioning for as long as possible within realistic limitations.

— For **the aged patient in residence** who may never be discharged to a home setting, patient-care goals (audit outcome criteria) may be established for timed intervals (two, four, six, 12 weeks and six months). See Recommended References, "Guidelines . . . " by ANA. For convenience, goals have been combined in this guide. For additional nursing actions and information, see NCPGs #2:33, "The Aged Patient: Physiology of Aging," #2:26, "The Aged Patient: Common Behaviors," and #2:27, "The Aged Patient: Transition to Communal Living."

— Determine if your staff and colleagues have unresolved fears of aging, disability, dependency, and death that are affecting their patient care. Work with a psychiatric nurse counselor to explore feelings and suitable coping mechanisms. *Genuine* respect and affection for the aged are essentials for geriatric nurses.

Specific Considerations, Potential Patient Outcomes, and Nursing Actions:

1) Maintenance of Adequate Biophysical Status Within Age and Disease Limitations (Skin Integrity, Nutrition, Elimination, Exercise, Rest, and Cardiopulmonary Function)	The patient will perform some activities of daily living (ADL) with minimal necessary assistance; the patient will maintain normal, warm, moist skin and mucous membranes; the patient will have a minimum fluid intake of 1500 ml/day, an output of at least 900 ml/day, and at least one bowel movement every four days; the patient will attain and maintain desired weight; the patient will participate in exercise and rest periods daily, ambulating with assistance as necessary; will sleep at least six hours nightly (preferably without sedation); the patient will have clear lungs and normal vital signs: — record vital signs & I&O at least QD & weight a least 2 x/week; — offer 6 small feedings daily of nutritionally balanced foods & fluids to achieve goals for fluid intake & output; — arrange for pt. to have eyeglasses, hearing aid, false teeth, & other assistive devices for ADL PRN; — supervise medication consumption (kind, time, & amount); know side effects of drugs given & carefully observe & record pt. responses to all medications & treatments; — provide range-of-motion exercises at least QD (see NCPG #1:47); if ambulatory, use exercises as suggested in NCPG #2:32, "The Aged Patient: Exercises for Patients Over 65;" for additional nursing actions & information, see NCPG #2:45, "Hazards of Immobility;" — keep skin clean, dry, & free of surface irritants or pressure impeding circulation; see NCPG #4:42, "Decubitus Ulcer Care: Prevention and Treatment."
2) Maintenance of Adequate Psychologic Status Within Age Disease Limitations	The patient will regain and maintain contact with reality; the patient will be oriented to time/place/person; the patient will appear less withdrawn and apathetic, interacting voluntarily with others and with environment in socially appropriate ways; the patient will make some decisions and choices related to own care and activities and will reminisce to integrate life experiences: — get pt.'s attention before speaking; say name, wait for eye contact, speak slowly, distinctly, & loud enough to be heard; turn off radio, TV, & shut out other distractions;

(Orientation, Interaction, Interest, Motivation, Decision Making, Sense of Identity, and Self-Worth)	— use a voice tone that indicates sincerity, sensitivity, respect, & acceptance; — give pt. choices when possible, but avoid meaningless, unnecessary changes (room, roommate, decor, routines, etc.), which are often upsetting to OBS pts.; — have pt. do for self what s/he can, for as long as able; nevertheless, be readily accessible & willing to help with dressing, feeding, ambulation, & ADL PRN; consider safety & pt. capabilities, not just your own time, convenience, or workload; expect neither too little nor too much; keep nursing care plan realistic; explain this approach to family & friends so consistency toward pt. can be preserved; — observe, describe, & record common behavior patterns of pt.; identify cues that trigger adverse reactions & plan to avoid or control these; note whether this pt. is agitated by certain persons, topics of conversation, or situations; recognize that episodes of paranoia, aggression, temper tantrums, delusions, anxiety, despondency, rigid orderliness, fears, fantasies, apathy, stubbornness, & other behaviors might occur from time to time; know that medication (tranquilizers usually) can control much asocial, difficult-to-handle behavior & need to be considered for the safety & peace of mind of family who must care daily for these pts.; when sufficient numbers of skilled geriatric personnel are available to work with pt., medication dosages can be reduced; — answer questions repeatedly PRN, using short, simple sentences; demonstrate nonverbally to reinforce verbal communication; build on the sensible statements of the pt. to strengthen reality-based conversation; — provide hourly orientation to time/place/person; use clocks, calendars, signs, pictures, & written reminders; put pt.'s picture & name (big letters) on the door to room & on bed; — interview family & friends to identify successful coping mechanisms previously used by pt. for anxiety, depression, stress, etc.; attempt to incorporate their usage with necessary modifications; — use concrete symbols (photographs, tangible creations, & products) of pt.'s past to strengthen & reassure pt.'s sense of continuity of self (now threatened with brain deterioration); — encourage pt. to review past in order to remember & savor happy events, friendships, trips, achievements, etc.; even if content of reminiscences produces sadness, resentment, or angry outbursts, there is value in ventilation & working through those feelings before changing subject to a more pleasant one; — help family & friends so they will not withdraw from the pt.; guide & help them to understand & accept the pt.'s behavior, while at the same time helping them to work through their feelings of helplessness, anger, depression, love, & guilt; help them prepare for the pt.'s return home (if applicable) by raising questions, considering solutions, exploring alternatives, & deciding on a goal & plan of action that meets mutual needs;

- show you care by providing small gifts such as a flower, a favorite food or drink, a picture of a special pet or friend; use touch therapeutically *if* you feel comfortable in doing so;
- celebrate special events in pt.'s life (birthdays, anniversaries, religious days); observe customary national holidays with parties, decorations, special refreshments, & entertainment;
- utilize volunteers to visit or write letters for pt., to show films, hold concerts, or entertain, to take pts. for outings on grounds or in neighborhood, etc.; respect the pt.'s privacy (space, time, possessions);
- arrange for some kind of meaningful occupational therapy (simple repetitive activities such as clipping coupons, packaging items, stuffing envelopes, etc.);
- try carefully planned music as therapy for relaxation, mood lifting, sensory stimulation, or as a vehicle for communication & not just as a monotonous alternative to background noise;
- for additional nursing actions & information, refer to NCPGs #3:33, "The Aged Patient: Reality Orientation," #3:34, "The Aged Patient: Resocialization," & #4:35, "The Aged Patient: Remotivation."

Discharge Planning and Teaching Objectives/Outcomes

1) (Patient/Family/Significant Other) Expresses understanding of chronic disability and the medical regimen prescribed; indicates a willingness to follow a written program of activities for reality orientation, resocialization, and remotivation.
2) Recognizes need for ongoing medical and nursing supervision and consultation. Has name and phone number of attending physician, community health nurse, and available community resource groups (Meals-on-Wheels, Senior Citizen Self-Help groups)

Recommended References

"The Aged Patient: Common Behaviors." *NCP Guide #2:26*, 2nd Ed., Nurseco, 1980.
"The Aged Patient: Exercises for Patient Over 65." *NCP Guide #2:32*, 2nd Ed., Nurseco, 1980.
"The Aged Patient: Physiology of Aging." *NCP Guide #2:33*, 2nd Ed., Nurseco, 1980.
"The Aged Patient: Reality Orientation." *NCP Guide #3:33*, 2nd Ed., Nurseco, 1983.
"The Aged Patient: Remotivation." *NCP Guide #4:35*, 2nd Ed., Nurseco, 1983.
"The Aged Patient: Resocialization." *NCP Guide #3:34*, 2nd Ed., Nurseco, 1983.
"The Aged Patient: Transition to Communal Living." *NCP Guide #2:27*, 2nd Ed., Nurseco, 1980.
"Being Old is not the Same as Being Ill," by M. Dolarn. *Nursing 80*, April 1980:41, 42.
"Decubitus Ulcer (Pressure Sore) Care: Prevention and Treatment." *NCP Guide #4:42*, 2nd Ed., Nurseco, 1983.
"Hazards of Immobility." *NCP Guide #2:45*, 2nd Ed., Nurseco, 1980.
"Hope and Flexibility—Your Keys to Helping OBS Patient," by K. Richardson. *Nursing 82*, June 1982:65-69.
"Range of Motion Exercises." *NCP Guide #1:47*, 2nd Ed., Nurseco, 1980.
"The Patient with Alzheimer's Disease." *NCP Guide #5:02*, Nurseco, 1981.

The Aged Patient: Remotivation

Definition: Remotivation is a type of nursing therapy that continually stimulates the patient to engage in activities for the productive use of time, for creative use of energy, and for restoration of desire to enjoy life more fully.

LONG TERM GOAL: The patient/client will actively engage in activities designed to further own knowledge, physical or mental fitness, or services to self or society; the patient will communicate satisfaction, pleasure, and pride of achievement at conclusion of selected activities.

General Considerations:

— Only **patients in touch with reality,** who have successfully achieved goals of resocialization therapy, should be considered for progression to a remotivation program.

— **Remotivation programs** incorporate, but are not limited to, therapeutically designed, individualized programs of rehabilitation (occupational, vocational, educational, recreational and/or physical therapy). They are used for brain-damaged or severely handicapped persons, but are more commonly employed for the aged patient.

— Refer to NCPGs #3:33,"The Aged Patient: Reality Orientation," and #3:34, "The Aged Patient: Resocialization," for essential basic information that a nurse should use before planning a remotivation program. To be effective, nurses also need a fundamental understanding of the aged patient. See NCPGs #2:33, "The Aged Patient: Physiology of Aging," #2:26, "The Aged Patient: Common Behaviors," and #2:27, "The Aged Patient: Transition to Communal Living."

— **Remotivation therapy** aims to provide meaningful activities that are geared to stimulate interest and participation. People need to feel involved in personal, loving, caring, and understanding relationships and to do purposeful activity for which they are recognized and appreciated. To be most effective, programs must be planned around individual likes, dislikes, capabilities, and limitations.

— **Nursing responsibilities** include initiating and maintaining an individually designed remotivation program, as well as respecting the need for and making an effort to provide privacy, undisturbed silence, meditation, prayer, or thoughtful reflection, for elderly patients.

Specific Considerations, Potential Patient Outcomes, and Nursing Actions:

1) Alteration in Achievement Orientation (Loss of Achievement Orientation; Feelings of Uselessness; Lethargy and Lack of Motivation)	The patient will demonstrate an interest and desire to participate in meaningful learning or doing activities; the patient will express feelings of satisfaction, pleasure, and accomplishment upon conclusion of remotivation sessions: — portray a positive, enthusiastic attitude when discussing tentative plan with pt. & family; encourage them to express their goals, interests, & feelings; work out a simple plan to achieve realistic goals jointly set by you & family; — if pt. will work or learn in a group setting, establish a friendly climate of warmth & acceptance in which all members feel welcome, needed, & recognized for their participation; talk to the whole group, redirect questions, give feedback, & help members to share information with each other; — know that having a group-directed, relaxed work or study session does not mean that the nurse/therapist is unprepared or uninformed, or that the session is completely informal without a goal or a well outlined plan; — let pts. choose from a list of *specific* topics *after* selecting a general interest area (such as health, safety, nutrition, art, music, politics, gardening, etc.); — as members of the group gain knowledge, skill, & confidence, encourage each of them in turn (when ready) to select topics, provide supplies or visual aids, read or give presentation, demonstrate a skill, or help others to grow within the group; — utilize group games (e.g., Bingo, card games), herb or flower planting activities, preparation of holiday or birthday gifts & decorations, arts & crafts to develop muscle coordination, new skills, & opportunities for socialized learning; — for teaching suggestions, refer to NCPGs #1:48, "Teaching Patients: General Suggestions," & #1:50, "Teaching Patients: Specific Plan for Skills and Procedures;" — evaluate & document progress or change in pt.'s knowledge, behavior, & attitudes; remember, effects are often short-term unless remotivation sessions are continually ongoing & constantly reinforced with new ideas as well as repetition of knowledge & skills already gained.

2) Alteration in Life Adjustment (Inadequate Integration of Life's Experiences; Unresolved Conflicts; Unexpressed Fears, Feelings of Helplessness, Hopelessness)	The patient will talk about past life experiences in order to create a desire to become more actively involved in facing life's present problems: — know that talking about past experiences can help pt. establish rapport, identify successful coping mechanisms & strengths, & rekindle interest; — encourage pt. to identify own strengths ("Tell me something you did that made you proud."), to tell about happiest period of life, to express dissatisfactions (with the younger set, or with present society/government/economy, etc.), to describe what s/he feels made life most worthwhile, to tell about philosophy of life/death/God/man, to talk about family, holiday celebrations, favorite foods, entertainers, sports, & sports figures; — examine content of reminiscing sessions to identify possible fears, weaknesses, losses, regrets that may have a bearing on present perceptions, attitudes, opinions, or behavior; do not probe for details, nor offer interpretations; reinforce positive aspects; — calmly offer support by your presence & quiet attentiveness if pt. expresses angry outbursts, disappointment, resentments, vindictive or paranoid statements; do not attempt to quell the tirade or reassure prematurely, but allow the ventilation for its healing benefits; *then* redirect reminiscences to more positive topics; — encourage pts. to talk about something funny that happened to them long ago; use humorous incidents to relax tensions & feelings of discomfort, to restore a sense of perspective, not to avoid discussing painful stories; — arrange for roommates or agemates who can share memories of similar eras; — lead a discussion group that follows a sequence of life-cycle events; — use photographs, scrapbooks, old letters, & memorabilia to jog storytelling; play songs, lead a sing-a-long, cook or serve foods that pts. haven't had for a long time; discuss special historic events or sports achievements & persons to stimulate memories.

Discharge Planning and Teaching Objectives/Outcomes

1) (Patient/Family/Significant Other) Understands medical regimen and indicates a willingness and confidence to follow it.
2) Expresses awareness of needs for purposeful activity and has stated s/he will continue those things discovered to be most satisfying and productively successful.
3) Recognizes that regression is possible and will seek help from community health nurse, senior citizen group, or other known neighborhood resources when developing signs of lethargy, loss of interest and motivation, or feelings of uselessness and helplessness.

Recommended References

"The Aged Patient: Common Behaviors." *NCP Guide #2:26*, 2nd Ed., Nurseco, 1980.
"The Aged Patient: Physiology of Aging." *NCP Guide #2:33*, 2nd Ed., Nurseco, 1980.
"The Aged Patient: Reality Orientation." *NCP Guide #3:33*, 2nd Ed., Nurseco, 1983.
"The Aged Patient: Resocialization." *NCP Guide #3:34*, 2nd Ed., Nurseco, 1983.
"The Aged Patient: Transition to Communal Living." *NCP Guide #2:27*, 2nd Ed., Nurseco, 1980.
"Fear of Loss and Attachment," by C. Carter and D. Galliano. *Journal of Gerontological Nursing*, June 1981:342-349.
"Movement, Music, and Remotivation with the Regressed Elderly," by W. Needles and M. Baer. *Journal of Gerontological Nursing*, September 1982:497-503.
"Nursing Intervention in Support of Reminiscence," by M. Ryden. *Journal of Gerontological Nursing*, August 1981:461-463.
"Psychosocial Issues in Nursing Care of the Aged," by I. Burnside. *Journal of Geronotological Nursing*, November 1981:689-em-693.
"Reminiscing Psychotherapy with Aging People," by K. King. *Journal of Psychosocial Nursing and Mental Health Services*, February 1982:21-25.

The Patient with an Antisocial Personality

Definition: A cluster of personality characteristics manifested by deeply ingrained, basically unsocialized behavior; formerly known as sociopathic or psychopathic personality.

LONG TERM GOAL: The patient will recognize and observe limits in interactions with others.

General Considerations:

— **Characteristics:** The antisocial individual does not tolerate frustration, feels little guilt, and does not change behavior because of punishment. Though this person often has an outwardly pleasing, charming personality, s/he is loyal only to own self, has no close personal relationships, and "uses" or manipulates other people and events for own motives. There is a tendency to blame others for the same behavior; has never learned to give, only to take. The antisocial individual does not see self as mentally ill and infrequently presents self for treatment; usually hospitalized for treatment of other disorders, to withdraw from alcohol or drugs, or as result of a court order for psychiatric evaluation or treatment. Described as selfish, irresponsible, impulsive, and callous; repeatedly in conflict with society, and often with the law.

— **Treatment** usually consists of applying external controls to limit the acting-out behavior; antisocial behavior patterns are difficult to alter and respond poorly to treatment. Long-term psychotherapy has had the most success in changing behavior patterns, but relatively few patients remain in psychotherapy because of expense, time involved, and poor motivation and insight.

— **Nursing responsibilities** include reinforcing reality, preventing manipulation of self and others by patient, protecting other patients and self from this patient, and health teaching as needed.

Specific Considerations, Potential Patient Outcomes, and Nursing Actions:

1) Manipulation — The patient will recognize and observe limits in interactions with others:

— be aware that staff commonly experience uncomfortable feelings of anger, helplessness, frustration, defensiveness, etc., when working with these pts.; openly discussing & acknowledging these feelings with other staff can lead to control of them, thus making one less susceptible to being manipulated; refer to NCPG #1:29, "The Patient Displaying Manipulation;"

— observe closely pt.'s behavior & interactions with staff & other pts.; assess the meaning & understanding of the behavior to the pt. & validate with pt. & other staff; hold a staff conference to discuss, set, & inform all staff of approaches & limits for this pt.;

- be aware of other pts. who could easily be affected by pt. (used, hurt) & intervene PRN; work with both pts. on appropriate alternatives to respond to each other; if antisocial pt. refuses to cooperate, separate from rest of unit for time out; state firmly that limits will be set on behavior & that people & situations will not be used for one person's motives; make contract with pt. that states specific cause & effect, such as, "If you take Mr. H's cigarettes, you will not be allowed in the day room when he is there;" follow through on contract on all shifts; *be consistent*;
- review requests made by pt. with other staff before permission is granted or denied; do not make "on-the-spot" decisions if possible; remember that this pt. is often an expert at pitting 1 staff member against another (recreating the family triangle & s/he is the center of attention); staff must present a united front to the pt.;
- give attention to pt. when s/he is not manipulating; reinforce positive behavior (often the only attention pt. gets occurs after s/he "acts out" or manipulates); set reasonable goals with pt.; reinforce positive efforts to reach them;
- explanations, discussions should be short & simple since long, complex ones can be another aspect of manipulation;
- know that this pt. may refuse to recognize own inappropriate or manipulative behavior; it is more effective to change the subject or leave the situation than to argue or try to convince him/her;
- be aware that patient may use tears, lies, threats to get what s/he wants; limits must be followed by all staff members & may be lifted as pt. shows s/he can handle responsibility;
- know that pt's. demands may be endless; be firm &, most important of all, be consistent.

2) Difficulty with Social Relationships

The patient will strengthen ability to relate to others in socially acceptable ways:

- assess & help pt. define problem areas in social relationship, e.g., blames others, lack of concern for others;
- encourage pt. to discuss this problem area in group therapy & to ask others why they reject him/her (if true);
- practice social skills, use role-playing; give positive reinforcement for positive behavior.

3) Acting Out or Violent Behavior

See NCPG #4:40, "The Patient Who is Violent."

Discharge Planning and Teaching Objectives/Outcomes:

1) (Patient/Family/Significant Other) Can cite some limits to interactions with others.
2) Has demonstrated ability to comply with social mores and to behave within socially acceptable limits at least part of the time (to an increasing amount).
3) Indicates a willingness to continue mental health therapy in some form that is presently available and potentially helpful.

Recommended References

"Behavior Modification." *NCP Guide #5:37*, Nurseco, 1981.

"Hospital Treatment of Borderline Patients," by B. Mark. *Journal of Psychiatric Nursing and Mental Health Service*, August 1980:25-310.

"The Manipulative Patient," by M. McMorrow. *American Journal of Nursing*, June 1981:1188-90.

"The Patient Displaying Manipulation." *NCP Guide #1:29*, 2nd Ed., Nurseco, 1980.

"The Patient Experiencing Powerlessness." *NCP Guide #5:34*, Nurseco, 1981.

"The Patient Who is Violent." *NCP Guide #4:40*, 2nd Ed., Nurseco, 1983.

"Treatment of the Acting Out Borderline Patient in Private Practice", by S. Lego. *Clinical and Scientific Sessions* NP#-59), Kansas City, MO: American Nurses Association, 1979:333-341.

The Patient with a Developmental Disability: Mental Retardation (in an Acute Setting)

LONG TERM GOAL: The patient will maintain admission levels of functioning within limitations imposed by current illness.

General Considerations:

— Read NCPG #4:38, "The Client with a Developmental Disability: Mental Retardation (in a Residential Setting)."

— **Incidence of disease/accidents:** retarded persons get their share of acute and chronic diseases and accidents. Certain handicaps are often associated with mental retardation (MR), such as cerebral palsy and epilepsy. An HEW study in 1971 showed that nearly 88% of MR individuals have one additional handicap. Because of these allied health problems, MR patients are prone to complications of normal illnesses such as upper respiratory problems and other secondary infections.

— **Nursing responsibilities** include respecting and considering the retarded person's life experience, years lived, IQ, and mental age (MA); assessing abilities and limitations in activities of daily living (ADL), social skills, knowledge/attitudes about MR, medical diagnosis, and regimen with both patient and family/guardian/significant other (SO); providing information about regional and national MR organizations as needed and wanted; providing care dictated by medical diagnosis and regimen and adapted to accommodate this patient's particular needs and abilities. In addition, nurses need to be exceedingly patient with the MR client and will find it necessary to explain their duties frequently, in an easy-to-understand fashion.

Specific Considerations, Potential Patient Outcomes, and Nursing Actions:

1) Activities of Daily Living (ADL)

The patient will maintain admission levels of functioning (state them) in ADL:

— assess pt.'s usual level of ADL by asking pt./family/SO, & adapt these to hospital routine PRN; it is desirable to maintain former patterns & habits in order to minimize pt.'s anxiety during the period of acute illness or trauma;

— be aware that some regression may occur due to taking on sick role during acute or chronic illness; minimize this by encouraging self-care & work with pt. & family to maintain good health habits & self-care patterns;

— *dressing:* encourage pt. to dress self in own clothing; if hospital clothing is a must, some minor adjustments may help pt. to be independent; allow ample time for dressing & praise positive behaviors;

— *bathing & cleaning teeth*: help pt. set up convenient routine, using equipment used at home such as electric toothbrush, hairdryer; tactfully observe for cleanliness & assist only if necessary;

— *toilet procedures*: follow procedure used at home, using usual words & time schedule; may need to remind Q2H or get up at night; do *not* diaper;

- *nutrition:* assist pt. to choose foods s/he likes & can manage on diet as ordered; encourage self-help & health teach to attain understanding of well balanced diet, using simple terms, demonstration, & return demonstration of basic food groups, etc.; provide snacks;
- *sleep/rest:* explain hospital routine & assist pt. to relax during rest periods & sleep at night by following usual sleep routine with lights, snacks, favored objects, music, etc.

2) Teaching/ Learning Needs

The patient will be able to state/demonstrate (specify information/procedure) by (set a completion date):

- MR persons often have difficulty with verbal expression & vocabulary, thus behavior modification techniques are effective in learning new tasks, since little verbal exchange is required;
- use pt.'s own words or teach simple words/concepts; break concept/procedure into small components & allow pt. to practice/talk about each component, giving positive reinforcement & constructive feedback with each practice;
- know that MR persons are easily distracted, thus reducing their ability to concentrate on a specific task; this may lead to feelings of anger or frustration with subsequent self-injurious behavior such as slapping, biting, hanging of head, etc.;
- be creative in adapting pt.'s life experience to learning experience;
- health teach family/SO as necessary;
- see NCPGs #1:50, "Teaching Patients: Specific Plan for Skills & Procedures," #3:32, "Teaching the Parent/Guardian/Child," & #5:37, "Behavior Modification."

3) Medications and Treatments

The patient will accept and show understanding of reasons for medications and treatments by explaining them to nurse in own words:

- prepare pt. for procedures & treatments by explaining ahead of time what to expect & when to expect it, using words pt. understands, & asking pt. to repeat what s/he understands in own words;
- listen & learn what pt. expects & help correct misunderstandings;
- maintain uniformity in treatments/procedures & explain changes;
- give emotional support by staying with pt. during treatments/procedures;
- explain to pt. & family necessary information about each medication (name, dosage, time of administration, toxic effects to report); observe & chart observations; spot check pt.'s retention of information; health teaching should be simple, short, & relaxed.

4) Safety	The patient will comply with hospital safety rules and will ask for help when s/he needs it: — explain hospital routine, do's & don'ts, in simple, relaxed way, including use of call lights, siderails, O_2, other equipment PRN; have pt. repeat in own words to facilitate understanding; encourage to ask for help when needed; answer call light promptly; — assess need for & provide safety devices PRN: e.g., siderails, wheelchair, walker, etc.; — be aware that many MR pts. tend to put things in their mouth or do unpredictable things with loose objects; close supervision may be necessary.
5) Psychosocial Adjustment to Hospitalization	The patient will adapt to hospital setting and will develop and maintain feelings of self-worth: — respect & consider the pt.'s life experience & age regardless of IQ or retardation levels; do not treat the adult person as a child even though his developmental age is that of a child; — give positive reinforcement to self-help behaviors & socially acceptable attitudes & behaviors; praise healthy habits & attitudes; — facilitate expression of feelings & encourage pt. to share experience of hospital with nursing staff; — encourage questions; assign permanent staff to pt. if possible to build trust & rapport; — spend time & give support to family/guardian/SO; be attentive to information on ADL & health habits; health teach as necessary; discuss knowledge of regional & national MR services & provide addresses PRN; — be aware that pt. & SO/family/guardian/caretaker may have unusual degree of emotional dependence due to limitations of retarded person in daily life.

Discharge Planning and Teaching Objectives/Outcomes:

1) (Patient/Family/Guardian) Has received and can verbalize understanding of written set of instructions re medications, diet, exercise, treatments.
2) Verbalizes knowledge of all prescribed medications with name, dosage, administration times and directions, side effects.
3) Has information/appointment for next contact with physician.
4) Expresses knowledge of regional or national center for MR and has address(es) to contact them for services.
5) Has been evaluated for assistance (financial, vocational, home health care) and appropriate referral made.
6) Is aware that hospital/clinic is willing to collaborate with community agencies for reports, future care.

Recommended References

"Behavior Modification." *NCP Guide #5:37*, Nurseco, 1981.
"Behavior Modification by Parents in Home," by B. Haus et al. *Journal of Psychiatric Nursing*, August 1976:9-16.
"The Client with a Developmental Disability: Mental Retardation (in a Residential Setting)." *NCP Guide #4:38*, 2nd Ed., Nurseco, 1983.
"No Pity," by B. Barbieri. *American Journal of Nursing*, September 1976:1482.
"OR Nursing Care for the Retarded," by S. Roy. *AORN*, October 1976:672-678.
"Preparation of Mental Health Personnel for the Delivery of Mentally Retarded Services," by A. Hersh el al. *Journal of Community Mental Health*, September 1977:13-23.
"Teaching the Parent/Guardian/Child: General Suggestions." *NCP Guide #3:32*, 2nd Ed., Nurseco, 1983.
"Teaching Patients: Specific Plan for Skills and Procedures." *NCP Guide #1:50*, 2nd Ed., Nurseco, 1980.
"Understanding & Helping the Mentally Retarded," by G. Dodge. *AORN*, October 1976:679-684.

The Client with a Developmental Disability: Mental Retardation (in a Residential Setting)

Definition: Mental retardation (MR), as defined by the American Association on Mental Deficiency, refers to a sub-average general intellectual functioning that originates during the developmental period and is associated with impairment in adaptive behavior.

LONG TERM GOAL: The resident will learn to perform self-care activities with maximum independence for developmental level; the resident will develop and maintain feelings of self-worth.

General Considerations:

— **Manifestations of MR** include impaired learning, inadequate social adjustment, and delayed or lowered potential capacity for achievement.

— **Causes**

- *Before birth*: genetic variations (Down's Syndrome or Mongolism, Tay-Sachs), German measles or infection in mother during pregnancy, incompatible blood between mother and child (RH factor), glandular disorders, toxic chemicals, nutritional deficiencies, excessive drug use.
- *During birth*: birth injury due to long and difficult labor or very rapid delivery, abnormal position of fetus, difficult forceps delivery.
- *After birth*: inflammation of the brain from high fever due to childhood diseases, accident with trauma to head, glandular disturbances, inadequate stimulation in early childhood, postdrownings.

— **Levels of retardation** (classification system of American Association of Mental Deficiency):

- *Borderline/Level O*: IQ range 68 to 83, with a potential adult mental age (MA) of 10 years, 11 months to 13 years, 3 months; usually capable of marriage and being self-supporting, probably at a low socio-economic living standard.
- *Mild or Educable/Level 1*: IQ range 52 to 67, with a potential adult MA of eight years, six months to 10 years, 10 months; capable of working but needs some supervision in financial affairs. Fourth/fifth grade academic possibilities as well as vocational skills by adulthood; often has difficulty keeping a job in competitive market. School placement is usually in classes for the educable mentally retarded (EMR); can usually be maintained within a community setting.
- *Moderate/Level 2*: IQ range 36 to 51, with a potential adult MA of six years, one month to eight years, five months; first to third grade academic potential. Vocational possibilities usually at sheltered workshop or neighborhood job; school placement is usually in classes for trainable mentally retarded (TMR).

- *Severe/Level 3*: IQ range 20 to 35, with a potential adult MA of three years, nine months to six years; training goals are largely the self-help skills (toilet training, dressing self) with minimal independent behavior; school placement is usually in a developmental center for handicapped or TMR program; some are able to work in sheltered workshop.
- *Profound/Level 4*: IQ below 20, and adult MA potential is three to eight years and below, often accompanied by damage to CNS. Person may require total care.

— **Incidence:** one of 10 American families has an MR member; 70%-80% are in the borderline or mild (EMR) category; 20%-30% are moderately, severely, or profoundly retarded. The latter are most often cared for in residential institutions.

— **Factors found to promote residential self-sufficiency, adjustment, and mental growth** include: (1) clinical staff giving individual attention via affection, conversation, meeting physical needs; (2) residents having fewer contacts with MR peers and aides and more contact with non-MR persons and professional staff; and (3) staffing oriented to small groups with primary staff consistently responsible for same residents.

— **Treatment:** although the intelligence of the MR usually cannot be increased, much can be done to teach and reinforce socially desirable behaviors and attitudes, self-care activities of daily living, and to increase the quality of life.

— **Nursing responsibilities** include showing respect and consideration of resident's experience and years lived, as well as IQ and MA; working with interdisciplinary team to assess resident's needs, to plan and evaluate an individual program to help resident function at optimum level; observing and reporting physical signs and symptoms that might indicate a communicable disease, infection, etc.; and helping resident and/or family prepare for future and possible return to home or community placement.

Specific Considerations, Potential Patient Outcomes, and Nursing Actions:

1) Activities of Daily Living (ADL)

The resident will perform self-care in hygiene and grooming (and other ADL as appropriate for individual):
— assess ability to perform ADL including toileting, bathing, brushing teeth & hair, shampooing, shaving, nail care, dressing;
— identify areas of learning needs & teach activities to meet those needs.

2) Teaching/ Learning Needs

The resident will learn (state specific) skill/procedure by (set a completion date):
— assess learning needs & health teach in areas of self-care, family life, sex education, family planning, & VD counseling;
— know that MR residents tend to have decreased verbal skills & comprehension, & that problems with attention

span are acute in the severe & profound MR groups; use few words & more demonstration for short periods of time;

— choose a priority from the learning needs & focus on only one activity, skill, or procedure at a time; choose time of day when resident is rested & alert; choose an appropriate teaching area with minimal distractions;

— write out the exact steps of the skill the resident is to learn; break down to the most elemental components; arrange the steps in logical sequence (this is called *chaining*); always teach the chain in the exact order; use backwards chaining with MR, i.e., teach last step first and work backwards through entire procedure; e.g., 13 steps to wash & dry hands:

1) dispose of paper towel in container
2) dry hands
3) take paper towel
4) remove plug from sink
5) rinse soap from hands
6) scrub hands
7) put soap on hands
8) wet hands
9) place water in sink
10) place plug in sink
11) turn off cold water
12) turn on cold water
13) point to cold water tap on command

— teach only 1 or 2 steps of the chain in 1 session, or as you assess the resident can comprehend;

— reward ever longer chains (larger # of steps) until entire sequence is learned, then reward only completion of total task; have resident practice in different settings to promote transfer of behavior;

— guide, assist, or "walk" person through the actual procedure PRN, e.g., hold their hand while turning on faucet or picking up food with a spoon;

— urge resident to practice; reward any behavior that comes close to desired behavior;

— increase learning with use of praise & rewards that are important to resident, e.g., desired privileges, time with a friend or staff, music, TV, sugar-free gum, extra time out of doors; use food or candy as last resort as they tend to lead to overweight & dental caries;

— respond immediately if resident stops attending to lesson: say "no," ignore for 15 seconds, then resume teaching;

— bring reward/reinforcer to learner's attention PRN, e.g., hold gum at eye level & when learner attends, show next step & give the gum after s/he performs the step;

— be consistent, positive, & patient;
— when one skill is learned completely & adequately for that individual, repeat process with next skill or learning need.

3) Rest and Exercise

The *ambulatory resident* will preserve and improve independent functioning such as range of motion, strength, tolerance, coordination of ADL:
— work with PT & OT staff to assess, plan, implement, & evaluate an activity/exercise program to meet resident's needs;
— record kind & amount of exercise & ability to do same, as well as resident's reactions, tolerance, & coordination in ADL.

The *multiple-handicapped, non-ambulatory resident* will spend a major portion of waking hours out of bed, out of bedroom area, with some time out-of-doors daily; will have planned daily activity and exercise periods; will experience mobility and self-care whenever possible:
— work with interdisciplinary team to assess, plan, & implement daily activity/exercise schedule for resident; provide ROM or other exercise PRN; help resident to participate in group activities;
— observe resident's reactions to group activities; give positive reinforcement for positive behaviors, i.e., cooperation, support of other residents, enthusiasm, initiating interactions; work with resident to develop individual free-time recreational activities;
— encourage resident to work with & take care of own personal possessions such as games, arts & crafts materials, books, radios;
— refer to NCPGs #2:45, "Hazards of Immobility" & #1:47, "Range of Motion Exercises."

4) Nutrition

The resident will ingest adequate food and fluids and will eat in a manner consistent with developmental needs:
— supervise meal times PRN to ensure resident ingests an adequate amount of food; help resident to eat sitting at table in dining room, assessing areas where teaching is needed; give positive reinforcement for positive eating skills;
— use adaptive equipment PRN; chain components as in 2) above;
— chart food intake & percentage of meal eaten.

5) Medications and Treatments

The resident will ingest prescribed medications in a safe manner:
- when giving oral meds, ensure that resident swallows them;
- observe for adverse effects of meds & report any immediately;
- health teach effects of meds & self-administration as appropriate for MA;
- know that there seems to be a greater incidence of allergic reactions to drugs, food, & other substances among the MR; acquaint yourself with Rx procedures, explaining each step to resident; many people with MR have one or more handicaps & may need ongoing treatments.

6) Psychosocial Adjustment to Residential Setting

The resident will develop/maintain feelings of self-worth:
- respect & consider the resident's life experience & age regardless of IQ or MA levels; treat as an adult, even though developmental age may be that of a child;
- provide opportunities to spend time with a staff person or do small tasks, such as errands, etc.;
- give praise for efforts to maintain grooming, carry out ADL; give recognition to a new pair of shoes, haircut, dress, etc.;
- provide choices for resident so s/he has options, rather than a "you must do this now;"
- consider individual limitations & disabilities & find some things for resident to do at which s/he can achieve a degree of success;
- help resident vent anger & sort out the problem that caused it; frustration & anger often appear in MR residents due to poor verbal & communication skills; much patience may be needed to understand what resident is feeling;
- provide opportunities to learn simple money management skills & to be travel trained;
- provide information appropriate to level of functioning about family life, sex education, & appropriate peer relationships with members of the opposite sex;
- arrange for participation in programs inside & outside the setting for clients to have experiences that enable them to practice & utilize skills associated with developing peer relationships;
- distract pt. from potentially violent behavior into another activity; refer to NCPG #4:40, "The Patient who is Violent;"
- work with social worker & other staff to help resident's family develop constructive & personally meaningful ways to support resident's experience in the institution;
- work with family to prepare for resident's return home or community placement.

Discharge Planning and Teaching Objectives/Outcomes

See this section in NCPG #4:37, "The Patient with a Developmental Disability: Mental Retardation (in an Acute Setting)."

1) If a home or community placement is possible, (the resident) can carry out self-care activities (state them).
2) Has a plan for care of client as s/he gets older; plan is acceptable to client, family, and significant other.

Recommended References

"The Agonizing Decisions in Mental Retardation," R. Yeaworth. *American Journal of Nursing*, May 1977:864-867.

"Behavior Modification and Therapy in Mental Retardation," by N. Hyde. *American Journal of Nursing*, May 1974:883-886.

"Developing Sexuality Among People who are Retarded," by A. Pattullo. *Mental Retardation, Nursing Approaches to Care*. St. Louis: Mosby, 1978.

"Hazards of Immobility." *NCP Guide #2:45*, 2nd Ed., Nurseco, 1980.

Mental Retardation: Nature, Cause and Management, by G. Baroff. New York: Wiley, 1974.

The Mentally Retarded: Answers to Questions About Sex, by A. Attwell and C. Jamison. Los Angeles: Western Psychological Services: 1977 (an excellent reference for sexuality, VD, family counseling for MR).

"The Patient with a Developmental Disability: Mental Retardation (in an Acute Setting)." *NCP Guide #4:37*, 2nd Ed., Nurseco, 1983.

"The Patient who is Violent." *NCP Guide #4:40*, 2nd Ed., Nurseco, 1983.

"Range of Motion Exercises." *NCP Guide #1:47*, 2nd Ed., Nurseco 1980.

"Where Hope for Mental Retardation Grows Brighter," by I. Horoshak. *RN*, June 1976:39-43.

The Adult Victim of Rape/Sexual Assault

Definition: Rape is any forced sexual activity. The legal definition refers to forced, vaginal penetration. Other forced sexual acts may be referred to as sexual assaults.

LONG TERM GOAL: The victim will regain her emotional, physical, social, and sexual equilibrium.

General Considerations:

— **Incidence:** more than 82,000 rapes were reported in the US in 1980 (FBI statistics); it is believed that the actual number is three to 10 times that amount. The number of rapes per 100,000 females is 71—more than double what it was 10 years ago. Although men, women, and children are raped, most rapes and sexual assaults are committed by men against women.

— The **result of rape** for the victim is the disruption of her physical, emotional, social, and sexual equilibrium. The rape is a situational hazard and a true emotional crisis may or may not occur, depending upon the victim's coping mechanisms and available sources of support. The way a victim is treated in ER, by police, courts, family, can often be the "last straw" that pushes her into an actual crisis; refer to NCPG #2:31, "Crisis Intervention." The psychological impact is severe, may be long lasting, and is significantly affected by the type of immediate care the victim receives.

— In the past, research and attention have focused primarily on the rapist; now, due largely to efforts and research by women, the focus is on the victim and her ensuing disequilibrium.

— Many **myths** are perpetrated about rape but the **realities** are far different:

- *myth* Women "lead men on" and "ask for it" by their dress and behavior.
- *reality* Most rapes are planned by the rapist and are not provoked by dress or behavior. Ask youself how young children or 80-year-old women might have dressed or behaved.
- *myth* Most rapes are spontaneous and unplanned.
- *reality* Most rapists have observed their victim's living patterns and planned the attack.
- *myth* Rapists are usually strangers to their victims.
- *reality* Most rapists are in some way acquainted with their victims, either casually, or fairly well-known.
- *myth* Most rapes are racial and are usually done by black men against white women.
- *reality* Most rapes are intra-racial; one study showed that 70% of all urban rapes were committed by black men on black women.

- *myth* Rape is a sex crime.
- *reality* Rape is a crime of violence and power in which the rapist gets emotional, and usually sexual, gratification from physical dominance and control over a powerless victim.
- *myth* Rape is a nonviolent crime.
- *reality* Rape is a violent crime, usually carried out under threat of death.
- *myth* Many women will consent to sexual intercourse, then cry "rape" out of revenge or hysteria.
- *reality* Only about 2% of all rape and related sex charges are found to be false—about the same percent as other felonies.
- *myth* Women secretly want to be raped.
- *reality* Some women do fantasize about rape, but usually as aggressive sex, and not for what it really is: a terrifying, brutalizing, and humiliating experience. Rape is not sex by consensus.
- *myth* It could never happen to me.
- *reality* All women are potential rape victims, regardless of age, race, circumstances, dress, or physical attributes.
- *myth* Rape is motivated by sexual needs.
- *reality* Most rapists have other sexual partners, have normal personalities, and are much like most men you meet, only with a greater tendency to express violence and rage.

— **The Emergency Room (ER) experience** can be either a calming, supportive one, or one in which the victim experiences further injustice from the ER staff due to professional insensitivity and unhelpful attitudes:

- ER staff often question, "Was she really raped?" and put blame and responsibility on the victim. Frequently, this is because the staff person is made aware of own vulnerability to rape when confronted with a victim, and the situation is understandably anxiety-producing.
- Research shows that **typical reactions of rape victims** in ER are either "expressed," such as crying, laughing, nervousness; or "controlled," e.g., outward calm. If a victim is exhibiting the latter behavior, there is a tendency among ER staff to feel that she has not been raped, or is dealing with it so well that she needs no help.
- Staff often experience feelings of being overwhelmed by victim and not knowing what to do.
- ER staff should realize that the victim has just emerged from a terrifying experience and is not responsible for what was done to her; the rapist is responsible for the attack. When ER staff can understand this and act accordingly, they have an excellent opportunity to help alleviate the trauma inherent in the ER experience itself, to help the victim regain her equilibrium, and, potentially, to prevent future psychological problems.

- — **Goals of medical treatment** are to prevent infection, VD, and pregnancy, and to collect physical evidence.
- — **The ER nurse's responsibilities** include believing what victim says; providing basic crisis intervention; providing for immediate safety needs of victim; providing and assisting with medical treatment needs; collecting and preparing evidence for the police; providing community referral resources; being aware of own feelings and attitudes and their effect on contact with victim; and providing anticipatory guidance to the victim and family/significant other (SO).

Specific Considerations, Potential Patient Outcomes, and Nursing Actions:

1) Acute Physical and Emotional Reaction (Rape/Trauma Syndrome)

The victim will receive situational support from staff and be allowed to cope with situation in her own way; she will regain a measure of control over her life; she will receive appropriate medical treatment:

- — always provide a private examining room;
- — listen to what the victim is saying (this will help her regain control) & *believe* what she says (ER is not the place to be judgmental); acknowledge the assault, encourage her to talk, & be supportive of her (e.g., "It must have been a terrifying ordeal for you . . ."); express warmth, interest, respect, & a nonjudgmental attitude; allow open ventilation of feelings, especially anger at the rapist; be aware that this anger may be directed at staff;
- — ask her what is the most difficult thing for her right now & discuss it with her, refraining from giving advice of "You should have . . ." or "Why did you . . .?" (such statements will not be helpful);
- — if she says "It was my fault," or "I should have . . .," reinforce that the attack was *not* her fault, but the fault of the rapist, & that she did what she was forced to do in order to save her life (many victims "pay" the rapist for their life with the sexual act, then feel guilty, unclean, ashamed, self-critical);
- — encourage victim to express her feelings about the experience (usually of overwhelming terror), but do not dwell on the sexual aspects;
- — victim may not wish to talk and/or may look undisturbed, or seem to be coping extremely well; may be denying or minimizing the attack; allow her to cope in this way but tell her that at a later date she may experience feelings of anger, fear, or sadness, & that this would be a normal reaction;
- — do all interviewing sensitively & with consideration for victim's feelings; while it will be necessary (for court records) to know the explicit sexual acts involved, only *1* person needs to gather this information *once* (either MD or nurse); others can read it in the chart;

- — have a female staff member be with victim at all times, to be her advocate, especially during any examination or interrogation; if your hospital has a rape team, a member may fulfill this function; if victim asks for a female police officer, make all attempts to comply with request;
- — assess victim's ability to cope, i.e., what is her level of anxiety? her perception of what occurred? does she have available family/SO outside the hospital? what is her emotional response?
- — express your belief in her ability to deal with problems/decisions she will face in next few days; be sure she takes an active role in making & carrying out plans, e.g., reporting to police, returning to work, etc.
- — assist with collection of physical evidence (read NCPG #4:46);
- — if victim is alone, & she consents, call her family/SO & ask them to bring a change of clothes for her; if she has no one to call, develop a safety plan for her, e.g., transportation home;
- — provide her with information about available counseling services, option, rights, & follow-up treatments; allow her to use telephone to call crisis/rape center.

2) Reaction of Family/SOs to the Victim's Experience

The family/SO will verbalize an understanding of what victim has experienced; the family/SO will give client situational support:

- — assess family/SO's reaction to the victim's situation; be aware that they often tend to blame the victim, to be nonsupportive, & to isolate her; reinforce that the attack was not the *victim's fault or responsibility* & that it was a *terrifying* experience in which she was afraid she would be killed; that whatever her response to the rapist was, it was a decision made to try to save her life or prevent bodily harm to herself and/or to others;
- — family/SOs may feel they are responsible because they weren't there to protect victim & thus feel guilty & vulnerable; again, emphasize that the responsibility lies with the attacker;
- — assess & discuss with them ways they can be supportive to victim, e.g., by listening to & believing what victim says; encouraging & allowing victim to talk; helping victim to resume her usual life activities; not overprotecting her; letting victim make the decision to prosecute or not; not dwelling on the sexual part of the rape, but on the victim's *feelings* (usually ones of overwhelming terror); stress that victim needs to be held & stroked just as she would in any stressful situation, and not to withhold touch (otherwise they may reinforce victim's feelings of being unclean, ruined);

- share with them that it is typical that rape victims will have increasing fear & anxiety during next 48 hours & may want to talk at length about the experience; that victim may then "seem" to adjust, but may re-experience the feelings of the attack at a later date;
- tell them that the victim may not want to talk about the assault, & if so, they should not press her but continue to provide caring & support;
- tell them to work out with victim ways for her to *be* & *feel* safe, e.g., locks on windows, new lights, not walking alone at night, etc.; some action may need to be taken immediately, e.g., changing locks;
- assess SO's coping; often they are the ones to go into crisis & need a mental health referral for themselves; assess victim's equilibrium after she sees family/SO.

Discharge Planning and Teaching Objectives/Outcomes

1) Victim has someone to leave ER with, does not have to go home alone.
2) Has a referral and/or contact with a mental health counselor. Has resources or referral to a doctor/clinic for follow-up physical care.
3) Knows how to use prescribed medications, and symptoms/reactions to watch for.

Recommended References

"Evaluation of a Sexual Assault Treatment Center," by J. Bushnell. *Nursing Administration Quarterly*, Spring 1980:61–80.
"Evidence Collection: Rape/Sexual Assault." *NCP Guide #4:46*, 2nd Ed., Nurseco 1983.
"Improving Emergency Department Care of the Sexual Assault Victim," by S. Tolbert et al. *Annals of Emergency Medicine*, June 1980:293–297.
"The Patient Needing Crisis Intervention." *NCP Guide #2:31*, 2nd Ed., Nurseco 1980.
"The Patient Experiencing Powerlessness." *NCP Guide #5:34*, Nurseco, 1981.
"The Patient Experiencing Shame/Embarrassment." *NCP Guide #5:35*, Nurseco, 1981.
"Rape: the Process of Recovery," by D. Spema. *Nursing Research*, September/October 1979:272–275.
"Relief for the Rape Victim." *Emergency Medicine*, August 15, 1981:204–208.
"Sexual Assault Victims," by B. Moynihan. *Issues in Mental Health Nursing*, January/March 1979:87–101.
"Symposium on Emergency Nursing. The Role of the Nurse in the Care of Sexual Assault Victims," by B. Moynihan et al. *Nursing Clinics of North America*, March 1981:95–100.

The Patient who is Violent

Definition: Violence is any physical behavior that is destructive to self, others, or property.
Acting out is any aggressive/angry behavior short of violence and includes verbal and nonverbal threats.
Aggression is a state of inner tension causing some discomfort to an individual and energizing him to overcome his environment, often using gross motor behavior.

LONG TERM GOAL: The patient will develop new alternatives to deal with aggressive impulses.

General Considerations:

— **Principles and procedures** for control of aggression, acting out, and violence should be a part of every mental health facility's routine inservice training; review procedure for your facility.

— **A therapeutic milieu** adequately staffed by well trained and caring health care workers can prevent most violence.

— Each violent incident should be reviewed with a goal of improving patient care by identifying situations that contribute to violence and by evaluating and revising interventions.

— **Interventions** that decrease perceived threat and diminish feelings of impotence in the patient are usually most successful. The theoretical reason for this is that violence is a response to feelings of impotence and helplessness in the face of a perceived threat. This threat may come at the time of admission to a mental health facility: the patient may feel that his worst fear has come true, for he has lost control of his behavior and is "crazy" and being locked up. This may be accompanied by a marked increase in anxiety behaviors as he realizes that he must obey the rules or take the consequences. With a threat from within and a threat from without, a patient may respond with fight, flight, or freeze responses. He is not allowed to leave the hospital; he may flee to his room, which he must share with other patient, and he feels increasingly impotent. As anxiety and stress increase, the ability to reason decreases, and the patient responds more to isolated stimuli and less to the content of the situation. See NCPGs #1:20, "The Patient Manifesting Aggression," and #1:21, "The Patient Manifesting Anger," for interventions to prevent violence.

Specific Considerations, Potential Patient Outcomes, and Nursing Actions:

1) Immediate Response to Violent Behavior	The patient will cease any violent behavior: — allow pt. to remain in present position; give pt. space & keep some distance away; — observe pt. while placing self between pt. & door if possible; do not turn back to pt.; move slowly & deliberately;

— ask other pts. to withdraw & leave area; speak in a calm, quiet tone;
— identify feeling of anxiety: "You seem upset; I'm concerned you might hurt yourself or others here;"
— encourage verbalization rather than acting out: "What happened to make you so upset just now?" offer alternatives: "I'll walk with you and we can talk about this." "Let's walk back to your room and discuss this." "Let's have a cup of coffee and talk about it." "I'll stay with you while you hit the punching bag;"
— provide reassurance or support & set limits: "I want to help you control your behavior right now so that you do not hurt yourself or someone else."

2) Increasing Violent Behavior; Physical Restraints

The patient will tolerate physical restraints to prevent expression of violence:
— assemble equipment & staff; 4 staff members necessary to restrain average-sized pt.; if time available, staff should remove glasses or pens or other potentially harmful articles from their person; a blanket or sheet & soft leather arm & leg restraints may be needed;
— prepare a private room that contains a bed with a metal frame to which restraints can be secured; clear this room of other potentially dangerous items; hallway to room should be cleared of pts. & visitors;
— explain to pt.: "We're concerned about this behavior and we're going to help you control it now so that you don't hurt yourself or others."
— distract the pt. with blanket or sheet as if you were about to wrap him totally with it; during this attempt to distract, each staff member should take an arm or leg, raise pt. off his feet & place him face down on floor so that he loses his base of support for physically assaultive behavior; use good body mechanics & be aware of pt.'s body alignment to prevent injuries to staff & pt.;
— transport pt. to his room (each limb still carried by a staff member, with the legs carried from above the pt.'s knees); if necessary for control, carry face down; protect head; if necessary, 1 staff member can carry both legs;
— follow facility procedure for application of restraints; care should be taken to ensure that the restraints do not impair circulation or cause pressure to underlying nerves; *A PT. IN RESTRAINTS SHOULD NEVER BE LEFT ALONE*; stay with pt. & encourage to express thoughts & feelings about the incident; explore the situation that caused the pt. to experience increased anxiety & loss of control;
— remove all items from pt.'s clothing, especially potentially dangerous, sharp items, & matches;
— obtain MD's order for restraints prior to or immediately after emergency situation; if MD orders a parenteral medication, it may be given to pt. either at site of loss of control or after transporting pt. to room;

— take BP & pulse Q30 minutes & check extremities for signs of lack of circulation or pressure; offer snacks & fluids; give mouth care PRN;
— remove restraints as soon as possible when acute agitation subsides;
— allow other pts. who may have observed restraining & transporting to ventilate their feelings & concerns about pt. or their own potential loss of control.

3) Impulse Control

The patient will demonstrate increased ability to control aggressive impulses:
— see NCPG #3:35, "The Patient Experiencing Depression," sections (1) Sadness, Grief, Guilt, Anger, & (2) Self-Defeating/Destructive Impulses;
— explore violent episode or loss of control with pt.; identify why this act was done at this time; did this act have a "payoff" of decreased anxiety or relief of frustration?
— help pt. learn to identify the precipitating factors that led to anxiety & impulsive behaviors;
— assess pt.'s knowledge of own symptoms of increasing anxiety; health teach as needed; explore alternative, appropriate ways to deal with anxiety;
— explore pt.'s attitudes about expressing resentment, anger, frustration & other intense emotions; health teach appropriate expressions of resentment, anger, frustration, & assertive behavior; explore alternatives to over-control & withdrawal; use role playing & practice assertion techniques in group & individual settings;
— assess for knowledge & behaviors of problem solving & stress management (see NCPGs #5:47, "Problem Solving," & 5:49, "Stress Management"); health teach as needed, using pt. strengths to help with weaknesses;
— validate pt.'s appropriate responses to frustration, resentment, anger & anxiety;
— make contract with pt. that s/he will contact staff member when s/he feels symptoms of increasing anxiety & fears loss of control; plan with pt. for alternative behaviors to control aggressive impulses & express feelings in effective, nonviolent way;
— work with family/significant other so they may understand pt. & work with him to develop & support new coping.

Discharge Planning and Teaching Objectives/Outcomes

1) (Patient/Family/Significant Other) Can verbalize chain of events and feelings that have usually preceded a violent episode.
2) Has developed at least one new alternative for dealing with aggressive impulses.
3) Is able to express feelings in an appropriate way that is not harmful to self, others, or environment.

Recommended References
"Behavior Modification." *NCP Guide #5:47*, Nurseco, 1981.
"The Patient Manifesting Aggression." *NCP Guide #1:20*, 2nd Ed., Nurseco, 1980.
"The Patient Manifesting Anger." *NCP Guide #1:21*, Nurseco, 1980.
"The Patient Experiencing Depression (Psychiatric)." *NCP Guide #3:35*, 2nd Ed., 1983.
"The Patient Experiencing Powerlessness." *NCP Guide #5:34*, Nurseco, 1981.
"Perspectives on the Combative Patient," by D. Triconi et al. *Journal of Nursing Care*, November 1979:15–240.
"Problem Solving." *NCP Guide #5:47*, Nurseco, 1981.
"The Rageful Patient," by F. Clino. *American Journal of Primary Health Care*, January/February 1980:52–53.
"Stress Management." *NCP Guide #5:49*, Nurseco, 1981.
"Teaching Staff to Cope with Patient Violence," by B. Fein et al. *Journal of Continuing Education for Nurses*, May/June 1981:7–11.
"Training for Prevention of Assaultive Behavior in a Psychiatric Setting," by B.Oertz. *Hospital and Community Psychiatry*, September 1980:628–6300.
"The Use of Seclusion Rooms and Physical Restraints in the Treatment of Psychiatric Patients." *Journal of Psychiatric Nursing and Mental Health Services*, January 1980:13–16.

Assessment of Mental Status

Definition: An assessment of observable aspects of the patient/client's psychologic functioning.

General Considerations:

— **The mental status assessment** is a *method* of organizing clinical observations that provides a baseline for the patient's psychologic state; it also provides specific information to assist in establishing diagnoses, planning goals, interventions, and subsequent evaluation.

— In the practice of psychiatric nursing, the mental status is an integral part of the initial assessment. The complete psychiatric examination includes a physical and neurologic study by the physician, as well as a psychiatric history, which includes the statement of the problem, a careful identification of the present episode with the reason why the patient came in at this particular time, a personal history, and a family history.

— The mental status is a useful assessment tool in all areas of nursing practice. Additions to the initial assessment are made by daily observations in inpatient and day treatment facilities, as well as other community settings.

— The nurse may be the first to pick up symptoms of organic brain disease, alcohol or drug use, suicidal ideation, and inappropriate speech activity or behaviors; the patient can then be referred for a thorough medical and psychiatric examination by a physician.

— **The mental status examination** usually includes areas of (1) *appearance and behavior*, (2) *consciousness*, (3) *speech activity*, and (4) *thought process, content, and perceptions.*

Components of Assessment	**Examples of Abnormalities**
Appearance & Behavior	
Observe for *dress, grooming, & personal hygiene*; colors, makeup, condition of clothes; skin color & condition.	Inappropriate to age or place; condition of clothes unusual; unkempt appearance, unshaven, body odor; pediculosis or other unusual skin condition
Describe posture: erect, seated, horizontal.	Stooped, slumped; note open or closed posture
Describe gait	Shuffles, limps, fast, slow, akathisia
Describe motor behavior: ability to relax, level & pattern of activity, relationship to topics of discussion or activities & people around area.	Signs of anxiety: moist hands, restlessness or retarded movement, dialated pupils, carotid pulses visibly noticeable or bounding, pacing

Components of Assessment	**Examples of Abnormalities**
Appearance & Behavior	
Describe affect—facial expression & mobility: sad, serious, smiling, immobile, flat (no expression)	Grimacing, tremors, Parkinsonism, & bizarre movements of head & neck in phenothiazine reactions
Examine for scars & other marks.	Birthmarks, operative scars, needle marks, wounds, trauma on wrist, etc.
Note prostheses: eyeglasses, contact lenses, cane, dentures, etc.	
Note culture, growth & development tasks.	Inappropriate behaviors for culture, stage of growth & development.
Consciousness	
Determine orientation to time, place, & person by asking questions about the time of day, date, year, duration of hospitalization.	Disoriented to time, place, or person; stuporous, confused, clouded, unconscious
Use direct questioning if appropriate: "What day is today?" or "How long have you been here?	
Note sensorium: if patient is aware of his surroundings, his sensorium is said to be clear.	Unaware of surroundings
Speech Activity	
Describe quality: loudness, clarity, pitch, tone, inflection *Note quantity*: pace, volume *Assess organization*: coherence, relevance, circumstantiality	Slow, monotonous, flight of ideas; incoherent, circumstantial speech with neologisms (self-coined words); slurred speech, speech defect
Thought Processes and Content, Perceptions	
Assess feelings by verbal questioning such as: "How are your spirits? How are you managing? Do you get pretty depressed (discouraged, blue)? How do you feel about that? How low do you feel? How do you feel right now? What do you see for yourself in the future?	Important to assess for depression & suicidal risk; see NCPGs #3:35, "The Patient Experiencing Depression (Psychiatric)," #3:36, "The Patient with Manic-Depressive Psychosis", & #3:38,"The Patient who is Suicidal (on a a Psychiatric Unit)." Note evasiveness, hostility, anger, elation, tearfulness, distrustfulness, resentment, apathy, lack of openness & approachability.

Components of Assessment	**Examples of Abnormalities**
Thought Processes and Content, Perceptions	
Observe the way patient describes own history, symptoms, feelings; follow leads provided by patient's own words.	Incoherent, disorganized thoughts; blocking, irrelevance, loose associations, talkative, silent, aphasic
Ask appropriate questions such as: "What do you think about at times like this?" "Sometimes when people get upset, things seem unreal. Is this happening now to you?	Note indications of compulsions (repetitive acts that the patient feels driven to do), obsessions (recurrent, uncontrollable thoughts), doubting & indecision, phobias (irrational fears), free-floating anxieties (feelings of dread or impending doom; ill-defined dread).
Inquire about feelings of unreality, depersonalization (a sense that one's self is different, changed, unreal, has lost identity), feelings of persecution (a sense that the patient is disliked, persecuted, being plotted against), feelings of influence (a sense that others are controlling or manipulating patient), feelings of reference (a sense that outside events such as TV or radio are related to patient, communicating to patient, or about patient).	Feelings of unreality, depersonalization, persecution, influence, reference, delusions (false, fixed beliefs), illusions (misinterpretation of sensory stimuli), hallucinations (subjective sensory perceptions); assumes listening or watchful posture; attitude may indicate hallucations.
Assess for memory of recent events by asking about events in recent past; assess for retention & recall are by giving the patient several consecutive numbers and asking him to repeat them.	Poor recent memory in organic brain disease or high anxiety state Poor retention and recall
Ask patient to give a chronological account of his life to assess past memory. Ask about birthdays, anniversaries.	
Assess for attention & concentration: tell patient you want to test his ability to concentrate. Read a series of digits, starting with the shortest set and enunciating each number clearly at a rate of 1 per second; ask patient to repeat them back to you. If the patient makes a mistake, give a second try with a different series, such as: 8,5,6,3, or 3,5,6,8,2; or 9,7,6,6,3,2.	Poor performance of digit span is characteristic of organic brain disease; performance is also limited by mental retardation Unable to repeat at least 5 to 8 digits forward, or 4 to 6 backwards (the usual number).

Components of Assessment	Examples of Abnormalities
Thought Processes and Content, Perceptions	
Ask patient to repeat digits to you backwards. Ask patient to count backwards from 100 by 5s; note effort required, speed and accuracy of the responses.	
Assess judgment: ask about daily life of patient; note ability to compare thoughts, events, relationships, & draw solid conclusions. Ask "What should you do if you are stopped for a traffic/speeding ticket?" "What should you do if you miss the bus?	Unable to make comparisons of thought & events, understand the relationships, draw valid conclusions.
Assess abstract thinking: ask the patient to interpret simple proverbs such as, "A rolling stone gathers no moss," or "Don't cross your bridges until you get to them."	Concrete responses may indicate organic brain disorder, schizophrenia, low intelligence.
Assess insight: as assessment interview progresses, does patient show understanding of his present situation? How does he describe his problems or the cause of his present state?	Unaware of current problems or present situation; unaware of mental illness or abnormal behaviors. Unable to link cause & effect (these are associated with neurotic disorders.)

Recommended References

"Assessment of Psychiatric Patients," by C. Margolin. *Journal of Emergency Nursing*, July/August 1980:30–33.
"Mental Status Assessment . . . Programmed Instruction," by E. Harris. *American Journal of Nursing*, August 1981:1493–1518.
"The Patient Experiencing Depression (Psychiatric)." *NCP Guide #3:35*, 2nd Ed., Nurseco, 1983.
"The Patient who is Suicidal (on a Psychiatric Unit)." *NCP Guide #3:38*, 2nd Ed., Nurseco, 1983.
"The Patient with Manic Depressive Psychosis." *NCP Guide #3:36*, 2nd Ed., Nurseco, 1983.
"The Patient with Schizophrenia." *NCP Guide #3:37*, 2nd Ed., Nurseco, 1983.

Decubitus Ulcer/Pressure Sore Care: Prevention and Treatment

Definition: A decubitus ulcer is an area of skin where lack of blood flow has produced cellular destruction. Terms more commonly used are "pressure sore" and "bedsore".

GOALS: The skin will maintain adequate circulation to prevent tissue breakdown. If ulceration has occurred, the pressure sore will heal.

General Considerations:

— **Incidence and occurrence:** nearly 20% of the 39 million patients admitted annually to hospitals or nursing homes are "at risk" for pressure sores; of this group, one out of five will develop Stage II, III, or IV pressure sores (i.e., over 1.5 million patients yearly).

— **Classification** of decubitus ulcer/pressure sores:

- *Stage I*: skin area reddened, no break or impairment of integrity
- *Stage II*: skin bluish, mottled, or dusky-colored; superficial layers broken or blistered (vesicular)
- *Stage III*: subcutaneous layers broken down, no visible necrosis
- *Stage IV*: deep area of undermined tissue with layer of necrosis; bone, muscle, and fascia may be involved. "Eschar" is a thick, leathery, black crust of dead tissue, often covering an underlying necrotic process; when removed, "sloughing" occurs, i.e., drainage of "stringy" debris, it may be yellow, gray, or greenish color.

— **Causes:** inadequate circulation to an area of skin or friction damage to friable tissue. Most significant contributing factor is *prolonged pressure* on a body part where a bone is close to the skin surface and blood flow is restricted to that part for more than a few minutes. There is an inverse relationship between pressure and time, i.e., the greater the pressure the less time is needed to cause tissue compression, compromised blood flow, and subsequent ischemic pallor or blanching, followed by reactive hyperemia (redness). Another principle to remember is that the smaller the area of skin surface in contact with another surface, the greater pounds per square inch (psi) pressure is exerted on that skin area. Excessive heat or cold, moisture, and irritating substances are other factors that predispose toward and hasten tissue breakdown. Friction damage to skin occurs when patients are pulled up in bed or moved by pulling rather than by lifting. This horizontal sliding force is known as "*shear*," and also occurs with the patient's natural movements of heels or elbows on the bed surface.

— **Assessment of risk and susceptibility** to skin breakdown is decided by an evaluation of at least four basic variables:

- *general physical condition*, including nutritional and circulatory status: deemed "good," "fair," "poor," "debilitated," or "moribund and vegetative"
- *activity status*: ambulatory, walking with assistance, chairbound, bedridden (mobile or immobile, spastic or flaccid, partial or complete paralysis)
- *mental status*: alert, responsive, and cooperative; confused, depressed, or disoriented; stuporous or comatose
- *incontinence status*: absent (i.e., continent), occasional, consistent.

High-risk patients are those with a diagnosis of paralysis, diabetes, obesity, coma, malnutrition, dehydration, edema, anemia, spasticity, cirrhosis, malignancy or other debilitative disease that limits adequate mobility and tissue circulation. The relative risk probability and the type of disability are used to determine the number and kinds of intensive preventive measures to be implemented.

— **Prevention** of pressure sores should *begin* the first *minute* that patients are placed in a pressure-over-time relationship. Measures include:
- immediate use of pressure-relieving devices (static or nonmovable kinds like pillows, convoluted (eggcrate) foam cushions, gel pads, water beds, etc., and dynamic or movable types such as alternating pressure mattresses and Kinetic or Clinitron beds)
- movement of patient *as often as necessary* to maintain adequate circulation to all pressure points
- nutrition improvement (vitamin, mineral, protein, caloric, and fluid supplements)
- skin care (measures and products to keep skin clean, dry, soothed, protected, and intact; and
- effective teaching of nursing staff, patients, and their visitors (family and friends).

— **Treatment** aims to prevent further skin breakdown and to heal ulcerated skin by cleansing, disinfecting, debriding (with scalpel, with enzymes, or with mechanical means) and closing (by surgery and/or granulation).

— **Nursing responsibilities** include:
- accurately assessing the patient's potential for skin breakdown;
- developing a plan for prevention and treatment in consultation with primary care givers (including patient and family or friends);
- *supervising the implementation* of all preventive and therapeutic measures in the nursing care plan on a close, continuing basis;
- periodically evaluating results and progress;
- documenting pressure sore stage, location, size (in millimeters), appearance (inflammation, subcutaneous tissue

breakdown, undermining, eschar), drainage, odor, prevention and treatment measures (what, when, and how often), and results obtained (degree and rate of healing); and

- preparing a report of findings for sharing with staff and other colleagues through publication and seminars.

(*NOTE:* See Recommended References for suggested record forms or flow sheets.)

Specific Considerations, Potential Patient Outcomes, and Nursing Actions:

1) Pressure Relief

Prolonged pressure on bony prominences and other fragile skin areas will be avoided or relieved:

— inspect pt.'s skin at least Q8H; pay close attention to all bony prominences; document accurately & completely all areas of blanching or erythema that do not disappear within 30 minutes after source of pressure is removed;

— *according to need*, change pt.'s position hourly or at least Q2H; use a lift sheet to prevent trauma to skin due to shearing forces;

— maintain normal or neutral body alignment with pt.'s body weight evenly distributed; ascertain that supportive devices do not restrict circulation; position pillows or cushions effectively to provide comfort, alignment, & pressure-relief;

— utilize prone & semiprone positions when possible for more equitable weight distribution; know that even with equal distribution of weight & cushions, pressure on sacrum & buttocks is greater when in the sitting position than when in the recumbent position, therefore, do not substitute long sitting for equal periods of time in bed; it is the *change* in position that is valuable, not the position itself; also avoid Fowler's position in bed for longer than 30 minutes at a time;

— assess & relieve pressure produced by braces, prosthetic & orthotic devices, casts, traction, &/or indwelling tubes;

— teach pt. & visitors to help in observing skin changes & relieving pressure;

— to distribute & reduce pressure, use both static & dynamic pressure-relieving devices as appropriate; if you can't move the pt., put pt. on alternating pressure mattress, Kinetic, or Clinitron bed; use padded foot boards, foam or gel "boots" & "cradles" for heels & elbows; use silicone or gelatinous pads (such as Spenco Dermal Pad) for skin protection from casts, splints, braces, & prostheses; use natural or synthetic sheepskin pads, convoluted (eggcrate) foam cushions, liquid or gelatinous pads for protection of hips, sacrum, shoulders, other bony prominences;

— keep bed linens dry & free of wrinkles or ridges; use old, unstarched, soft cotton sheets to minimize skin irritation; do *not* place incontinence pads between skin & sheepskin or pressure-relieving pad, since this will trap moisture next to skin as well as defeat the purpose of pressure-relieving device.

2) Cleanliness All potential pressure sites will be clean, dry, free of surface irritants, and exposed to circulating air:

— whenever necessary (but at least BID), wash skin covering potential pressure sites with tepid water & mild soap (nonperfumed, nondeodorant type); use bath oils or moisturizers in bath water of all elderly or debilitated pts.; gently remove dry skin, caked powder, perspiration, crumbs, & bodily discharges; consider using commercial skin-care products (washes, creams, ointment) that emulsify dried feces, neutralize drainage, inhibit odors, promote healing, & provide a protective barrier;

— allow skin & skin barrier products to dry; provide freely circulating air by loosening bed linens/clothes & by leaving open to the air for at least 20-minute periods those heels, ankles, elbows, hips, shoulders, or coccyx otherwise cushioned or wrapped for protection; (*NOTE*: take care to avoid chilling pt.)

— seek to correct causes of incontinence while exerting efforts to watch pt. closely enough so that soiling accidents may be *promptly* remedied.

3) Circulation The circulation of blood to all potential pressure sites will be adequate to maintain tissue perfusion:

— gently massage potential pressure sites using mild astringents to dry & toughen skin;

— use heat lamps or portable hair dryers long enough to produce warmth & drying without causing harm (approximately 10–20 minutes); use safety precautions to prevent shocks & burns:

— provide active & passive ROM exercises to assist blood flow via muscular activity; see NCPG #1:47, "Range of Motion Exercises;"

— know that optimal healing takes place if hemoglobin is at least 12 & hematocrit is at least 36;

— consider CircOlectric bed, tilt frames, or kinetic (moving) beds to further promote circulation.

4) Nutrition The general physical condition and nutritional status of patient will be improved from previous levels:

— maintain fluid intake of at least 1800 cc daily; record I&O;

— increase daily intake of protein, calories, vitamins, & minerals to at least double or triple normal requirements, *especially* for pts. with Stage III or Stage IV ulcers (when tissue building is needed);

— use high-protein supplemental drinks or tube feedings when indicated;

— encourage visitors at pt.'s feeding or mealtime to promote appetite & to motivate consumption of more food, as well as to promote digestion & emotional satisfaction.

5) Treatment Measures: Stage I and II Lesions

The patient's stage I and II lesions will not progress to stage III & IV; the lesions will diminish in size and show evidence of healing by improved color and continued maintenance of skin integrity:

— utilize all applicable measures listed above for relief of pressure, promotion of cleanliness, & improvement of circulation, nutrition, & general physical condition;
— teach pt., family, visitors, & all nursing staff how to perform preventive measures as well as to assist you in necessary treatment of Stage I & II pressure sores;
— after cleansing lesion with mild soap & water, rinse with saline, & dry thoroughly;
— spray lesion(s) lightly with Granulex Spray Q shift;
— apply an occlusion-type dressing ("sealing is healing") with a commercial preparation such as OP Site, OP Dressing, Duoderm, Stomahesive, Bioclusive, Holliseal, Vigilon, Tegaderm, Bard Protective Barrier Film or Gel, or Spenco 2nd Skin;
— "picture-frame" surgical tape around edges of dressing (incorrect taping can cause blistering); write date on edge of dressing; observe BID; change when dressing becomes soiled, loosened, or is leaking;
— carefully document preventive & treatment measures & description of lesion.

6) Treatment Measures: Stage III and IV Lesions

The stage III and IV lesion(s) will steadily diminish in size and heal; any (both local and infection systemic) will be effectively controlled; granulation of healthy tissue will be successfully promoted:

— obtain weekly cultures of stage III & IV decubitus wounds (express fresh drainage, not what is obviously available); report results to MD, to infection control supervisor, & to unit charge nurse;
— obtain prescriptions for systemic antibiotics PRN & administer them correctly; know that topical & systemic antibiotics are useful only in selected cases;
— measure or estimate & record amount of necrosis, pus, odor, & inflammation; measure & record the length, width, & depth of lesion; photograph & label with lesion size & date; have 1 person obtain all indices on the same pt. to ensure consistency & accuracy; keep records up-to-date with twice weekly entries of all components measured;
— cleanse or irrigate wound with normal saline, hydrogen peroxide, povidine-iodine or Dakin's Solution; thoroughly rinse selected solution out of wound because it can inhibit the growth of newly formed tissue & impair the effectiveness of enzyme ointment; use whirlpool bath for pts. who have lesions that are large, deep, numerous, or otherwise inconvenient to irrigate adequately; dry wound with heat lamp or blow dryer;

— debride necrotic tissue, eschar, or slough by suitable method (surgically with scalpel or scissors; mechanically with whirlpool, Water Pik, gauze, or soft brush; or chemically with enzymatic agents such as Travase, Elase, Biozyme C); continue this treatment until all excess eschar & necrotic tissue is removed & there is granulation tissue forming; use products as directed, rinsing with saline or water; use sterile technique; keep enzymatic ointment away from healthy skin tissue to prevent irritation;

— to promote granulation, create a moist tissue environment; choose either "wet-to-dry" kerlix wound packing (time consuming & inconvenient) or use dextranomer (Debrisan) beads (which absorb tissue fluid);

— apply a semipermeable polyurethane dressing (e.g., Op-Site) "picture-framed" with surgical tape; write date of application on edge of dressing;

— observe BID; change only for loosened, soiled, or leaking dressing; leave in place for an average of 1–5 days, allowing serous fluid to accumulate under dressing; know that this moist environment accelerates granulation & epilthelization by allowing natural healing with body's leucocytes, plasma, fibrin, & epidermal cells;

— carefully document all preventive & treatment measures; supervise colleagues to ensure consistency of care & therapeutic effectiveness.

Recommended References:

"Assessment of Decubitus Ulcer Potential" (Form 101), "Decubitus Ulcer Flow Sheet" (Form 102), and "Position Chart" (Form 103). Whippany, NJ: Knoll Pharmaceutical Co., April 1977.

"Debrisan for Decubitus Ulcers," by S. Di Mascio. *American Journal of Nursing*, April 1979:684–685.

"Effects of a Liquid Copolymer Barrier in Preventing Skin Problems," by E. Shipes and I. Stanley. *Ostomy Management*, Spring 1981:19–23.

"Initial Nursing Assessment Form" and "Pressure Sore Flow Sheet." Columbia, MD: Dynamic Dimensions in Health Care (8729 Hayshed Lane, 21045).

"OP-Site for Decubitus Care," by M. Ahmed. *American Journal of Nursing*, January 1982:61–64.

"Pressure Sore Prevention—Aye, There's the Rub," by D. Feustel. *Nursing 82*, April 1982:78–83.

"Pressure Sores: What To Do When Prevention Fails," by G. Cannon. *Nursing 79*, January 1979:42–47.

"Range of Motion Exercises." *NCP Guide #1:47*, 2nd Ed., Nurseco, 1980.

"Saving Your Elderly Patient's Skin," by D. Mangieri. *Nursing 82*, October 1982:44–45.

"Stomahesive: The Astounding New Cure for Decubitus Ulcers," by M. Leeson. Cleveland, OH: Cleveland Clinic Hospital, (44106).

INITIAL NURSING ASSESSMENT FORM

Identify any patient at risk to develop pressure sores by assessing the six clinical condition parameters and assigning a score. Patients with a score of eight or above should be considered at risk to develop pressure sores. Initiate prevention protocol.

Choose the number for each parameter that applies to the patient's status. Total the six numbers to determine patient risk potential.

Clinical Condition Parameters			Score
General Physical Condition (health problem)	Good (minor)	0	
	Fair (major but stable)	1	
	Poor (chronic/serious—not stable)	2	
Level of Consciousness (to commands)	Alert (responds readily)	0	
	Lethargic (slow to respond)	1	
	Semicomatose (responds only to verbal or painful stimuli)	2	
	Comatose (no response to stimuli)	3	
Activity	Ambulant without assistance	0	
	Ambulant with assistance	2	
	Chairfast	4	
	Bedfast	6	
Mobility (extremities)	Full active range	0	
	Restricted movement	2	
	Moves only with assistance	4	
	Immobile	6	
Incontinence (bowel and/or bladder)	None	0	
	Occasional (less than 2/24 hours)	2	
	Usual (more than 2/24 hours)	4	
	Total (no control)	6	
Nutrition (for age and size)	Good (eats/drinks adequately—50%)	0	
	Fair (eats/drinks inadequately—50%)	1	
	Poor (unable/refuses to eat/drink—less than 50%)	2	
		TOTAL	

©Dynamic Dimensions in Health Care (8729 Hayshed Lane, Columbia, MD 21045). Reprinted with permission.

PRESSURE SORE FLOW SHEET

Circle location of ulcer on figure at right. Number ulcers if there are more than one. Document each.

Stage I: Reddened area. Stage II: Blister, skin break. Stage III: Skin break exposing subcutaneous tissue. Stage IV: Skin break exposing subcutaneous tissue, muscle and bone.

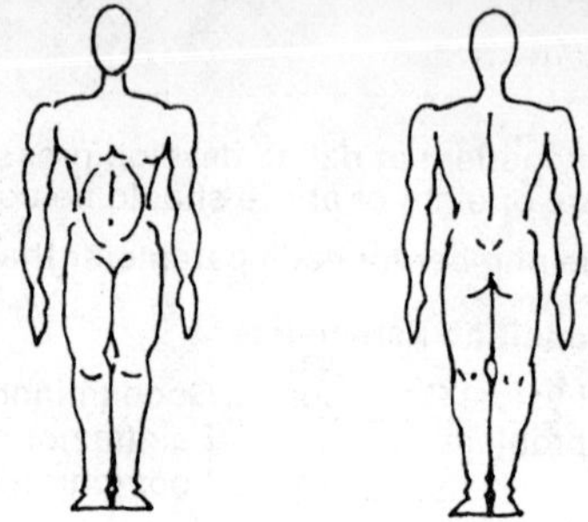

Assessment

Date								
Location								
Stage (I, II, III, or IV)								
Appearance*								
Size (cm.)								
Drainage**								
Odor***								
Inflammation								
Undermining								
Comments								

*pink = pink/red s = slough e = eschar **s = serosangineous p = purulent 0 = none ***0 = none m = mild f = foul

SIGNATURES

DATE				
11-7				
7-3				
3-11				

NAME PLATE

Management

Date												
Shift	11-7	7-3	3-11	11-7	7-3	3-11	11-7	7-3	3-11	11-7	7-3	3-11
Pressure Relief												
Skin Care												
Patient Movement												
Nutritional Care												
Patient Teaching												
Cleansing												
Treatment												
Comments:												

©Dynamic Dimensions in Health Care (8729 Hayshed Lane, Columbia, MD 20145). Reprinted with permission.

Diet: Fat-Controlled, Low Cholesterol

LONG TERM GOAL: The patient will demonstrate knowledge and ability to plan a fat-controlled, low cholesterol diet; the patient will ingest sufficient balanced nutrients and achieve high energy output through physical work and exercise to attain and maintain an ideal weight.

General Considerations:

- The major cause of coronary heart disease is atherosclerosis, which results in deposition of fatty materials within the arteries, predisposing them to clotting, obstruction, and ischemia. Atherosclerosis begins to develop early in life. The prevalence and extent of the atherosclerotic process can be reduced with proper diet, beginning at an early age, to control blood cholesterol levels.
- The average American ingests 600 mg of cholesterol daily; the recommended ingestion is 400 mg/day.
- Approximately 50% of the calories in the average American diet are derived from fat (should be 35%). Most of the fat ingested is of animal origin (saturated fat), rather than from plant sources (unsaturated fat). The ideal diet has a one-to-one ratio of polyunsaturated to saturated fat.
- **Nursing responsibilities** include teaching the patient/spouse/significant other (SO) the basic goals and principles of a fat-controlled, low cholesterol diet; assisting the patient to plan servings according to recommended calorie intake; providing satisfactory choices to patient, thus lowering resistance to diet; providing the patient with resource materials for accurate planning; helping patient plan own menus, critiquing and correcting them PRN; and providing tips on dining out, e.g., to order a la carte.
- **Guide to foods allowed or to be avoided on a fat-controlled, low cholesterol diet:**

Category and Recommended Daily Servings	Allowed	To Be Avoided
Milk Products		
2 Servings (1 serving = 8 oz)	Nonfat milk, buttermilk, yogurt; cheeses made from skimmed milk: non-fat cottage cheese, Sap Sago, mozzarella, hoop cheese	Whole milk, hard cheeses, ice cream, sour cream, commercial yogurt

Category and Recommended Daily Servings	**Allowed**	**To Be Avoided**
Fruits and Vegetables 4 Servings (1 serving = ½ cup)	All as tolerated; leafy green & yellow vegetables are good sources of Vit. A; citrus fruits, broccoli, cabbage & tomatoes are good sources of Vit. C	No restrictions unless calories are limited, then use only recommended amounts of potatoes, corn, lima beans; avoid butter or cream sauces on vegetables.
Bread and Cereals 4 Servings (1 serving of bread = 1 slice; 1 serving of cereal = ½ cup, cooked; 1 cup, cold)	Serve dry & cooked cereals with nonfat milk; macaroni, spaghetti, rice; bread (whole wheat, French, pumpernickel, white, rye), English muffins without shortening; saltine crackers, plain tortillas, rye crisp	Commercial pancakes, biscuits, cakes, crackers, doughnuts, coffee cakes, etc. made with whole milk & fat; commercial mixes
Meat, Fish, Poultry 2 Servings (4–6 oz)	Lean muscle meat, broiled or roasted. Use more often: chicken (without skin), turkey, veal, fish. Use less frequently: beef, lamb, pork, ham	Luncheon meat, frankfurters, organ meats, duck, shrimp, sausage, bacon, all heavily marbled & fatty cuts of meat; fried meat
Eggs	Whites as desired	Egg yolks: use only 3 per week, including those used in cooking.
Concentrated Fats and Oils (2-4 tbsp daily)	Margarine, liquid oils & salad dressings containing corn oil, soybean oil, cottonseed oil, sunflower oil, safflower oil, or sesame oil; read labels to identify ingredients. All nuts *except* cashew & commercially fried or roasted nuts. Freshly ground peanut butter; gravy made from fat-free stock	Solid fats & shortenings; butter; products with coconut oil, cashew nuts, mineral oil, peanut oil, olive oil; gravy & salad oils made with hydrogenated fats or olive oil; chocolate

Category and Recommended Daily Servings	Allowed	To Be Avoided
Desserts and Sweets (depends on limitation of calories)	Fruits; jellies; honey; puddings; cakes & cookies made with non-fat milk & without egg yolks; imitation ice cream made with safflower oil; angel food cake; gelatin; sherbet; low-fat yogurt; fruit drops, mints, jelly beans, & hard candy	Desserts made with whole milk, egg yolks, chocolate, coconut butter & animal fats; commercially prepared fried foods

Recommended References

A Guide for Weight Reduction; Recipes for Fat-controlled, Low Cholesterol Meals; Save Food Dollars and Help Your Heart. Dallas, TX: American Heart Association (7320 Greenville Avenue, 75231).

Nutrition and Diet Therapy, 4th Ed., by S. Williams. St. Louis: Mosby, 1981:611–617.

Drugs: Antileukemic

GOAL: To achieve complete remission (the disappearance of all abnormal cell forms in the bone marrow and peripheral blood) and to provide maintenance therapy once remission has occurred.

General Considerations:

— **Drug therapy** consists of three phases: remission induction, remission consolidation, and remission maintenance. This involves combinations of chemotherapeutic drugs to toxicity levels.

— **Combinations** vary among medical centers and from patient to patient, but all rest on basic tenets:

- cell sensitivity to chemotherapeutic drugs varies with the phase of the cell's life cycle; since only some of the cells will respond to certain drugs at any given time, treatment usually involves more than one drug;
- combination therapy allows use of a variety of drugs that have minimally overlapping toxicities and differing mechanisms of action, but are individually active against leukemia;
- toxicity is related to bone-marrow suppression and other side effects such as nausea and vomiting, and stomatitis.

— **Some combinations** that have proved effective and are frequently used are: (1) prednisone and 6-mercaptopurine; (2) vincristine and prednisone; (3) methotrexate and 6-mercaptopurine; (4) vincristine, methotrexate, 6-mercaptopurine, and prednisone; and (5) Ara-C, Daunorubicin, and 6-thioguanine.

— **Common characteristics** of antileukemic drugs include an affinity for rapidly dividing cells, including leukemic and healthy bone-marrow cells, hair follicles, oral mucosa, GI tract epithelium, lymph tissue, and gonads. All have toxic and side effects that require appropriate and prompt nursing intervention.

— **Nursing responsibilities** include assessing patient pretherapy for baseline data on vital signs, blood values, nutritional status, weight, skin, and mucosal status. After therapy is initiated, the focus is on monitoring the patient for early signs of side effects and minimizing these; working with the patient to accept the drugs in spite of the severe side effects; preventing complications related to side effects and preventing toxicity; reporting sharp, sudden decreases in WBCs (may indicate a need to decrease the drug); and carefully observing any IV administration to prevent extravasation of these drugs. Nursing management also includes teaching patient/family/significant other (SO) about drug dosages, actions, side effects, etc.

— Chemotherapeutic drugs used in the treatment of leukemia may be classified according to their mechanism of action:

1) **Alkylating agents:** effect a direct chemical interaction with the DNA in the cell, rendering it inactive and interfering with mitosis.

Example	Effective in Treating	Side Effects	Nursing Implications
busulfan (Myleran)	CML	Hyperpigmentation, pulmonary fibrosis, gynecomastia (with long use), cataracts, bone-marrow suppression	• Check for evidence of bleeding in urine, stool, mucous membranes; • watch for early signs of infection.
BCNU (Carmustine)	CML	N&V, transitory intense flushing of skin & conjunctiva	• Administer IV over 1–2 hour period; • Assess pt. for extravasation, which may cause burning or pain at injection site. • slow IV if pt. demonstrates intense flushing or redness of skin/conjunctiva.
chlorambucil (Leukeran)	CLL	Relatively nontoxic; some gastric discomfort, occasional urticarial skin rash, bone-marrow suppression	
cyclophosphamide (Cytoxan, Endoxan)	ALL, AML, & CML	Stomatitis, N&V, dermatitis, hemorrhagic cystitis, liver dysfunction, bone-marrow suppression, alopecia (hair loss)	• Cleanse mouth with moistened cotton swabs & nonirritating rinses. • Ensure a high fluid intake for 6 hours after Cytoxan is given in order to flush end products of drug out of bladder; N&V may make forcing fluids difficult; consult with MD regarding need for antiemetics. • Reassure that hair will grow back after drug therapy ends. • Check for evidence of bleeding in urine, stool, mucous membranes. • Watch for early signs of infection.

Example	Effective in treating	Side Effects	Nursing Implications
hydroxyurea (Hydrea)	AML, CML	Hyperuricemia with impaired renal function; give with caution to pts. with renal dysfunction.	• Monitor urinary output; ensure high fluid intake. • Check for exacerbation of postirradiation erythema.

2) **Antibiotics:** inhibit the formation of cell proteins.

Example	Effective in Treating	Side Effects	Nursing Implications
daunorubicin (Daunomycin)	ALL, AML, CML	Stomatitis, N&V, alopecia, red urine, menstrual irregularity; bone-marrow suppression	• Reassure that hair will grow back after drug therapy ends. • Be alert to signs of cardiac toxicity. • Give antiemetics PRN. • Explain to pt. that red urine is a side effect of this drug & not necessarily a sign of bleeding; • Watch for early signs of infection & bleeding.
doxirubicin (Adriamycin)	ALL, AML		

3) **Antimetabolites:** inhibit DNA formation thus blocking cell growth.

Example	Effective in Treating	Side Effects	Nursing Implications
methotrexate (Mexate)	ALL, AML, & CML	Renal toxicity, stomatitis, GI ulcers, diarrhea, N&V, photosensitivity, bone-marrow suppression	• May be given orally, IV, or intrathecally; if pt. complains of burning sensation with IV infusion, slow rate. • Provide mouth care with nonirritating rinses; oral ulceration is one of the first signs of toxicity. • Watch for signs of dehydration; record I&O accurately. • Dim lights in room PRN. • Check for signs of infection & bleeding.

Example	Effective in Treating	Side Effects	Nursing Implications
6-mercaptopurine (6-MP, Purinethol)	ALL	Liver dysfunction & toxicity; N&V, diarrhea, bone-marrow suppression; increased toxicity when given with allopurinol; use with caution in pts. with impaired renal function.	• Observe & report oliguria; force fluids to facilitate excretion of drug. • Be alert to early signs of toxicity (liver damage, diarrhea, & stomatitis). • Watch for signs of infection, bleeding. • Offer soothing mouthwashes; • Decrease dose if given with allopurinol.
6-thioguanine (6-TG)	ALL, AML, & CML	Similar to 6-MP but toxicity does not increase with allopurinol.	• As above (for 6-MP)
cytosine arabinoside (Ara-C)	ALL, AML, & CML	Stomatitis, esophagitis, N&V, diarrhea, skin rash, abnormal liver function tests, increased uric acid levels, bone-marrow suppression	• Administered IV, SQ, intrathecally; monitor for signs of extravasation. • Give 3–4 liters of fluid/day to increase uric acid solubility in urine. • Check for early signs of infection, bleeding. • Store unopened drug in refrigerator; when reconstituted, store at room temperature & use within 24 hours; discard hazy solution.

4) **Hormones:** suppress the growth of lymphoctyes.

Example	Effective in Treating	Side Effects	Nursing Implications
adrenocorticosteroid, prednisone	ALL, CLL	Euphoria, personality changes, increased appetite, susceptibility to infection, muscle weakness, headache, vertigo, sodium retention, menstrual irregularity, peptic ulcers, abdominal distention, diabetes; no acute toxicity	• Do not give on an empty stomach; give with food, milk, or an antacid. • Be alert to personality changes in pt. • Be alert to signs of fluid & electrolyte imbalance (see NCPGs #3:48 & #3:49); monitor blood serum levels; weigh daily & chart; record I&O accurately.

5) **Plant Alkaloids:** block the process of cell division (mitosis):

Example	Effective in Treating	Side Effects	Nursing Implications
vincristine (Oncovin)	ALL, AML, & CML	Constipation, diarrhea, abdominal cramps, sensory impairment, paresthesias in extremities; gait disturbances, poor coordination, stumbling; toxicity is related to cumulative dose.	• Given IV; ensure drug does not extravasate (it will produce necrosis). • For constipation, increase fluid intake; ensure that pt. has moderate exercise; offer fresh fruit daily; stool softeners. • For diarrhea, balance fluid intake to equal output; put on low-residue diet; cleanse perineal area well after each BM; check each BM for bleeding. • Check for tingling, numbness, weakness of hands & feet, foot drop, ptosis of eyelids; gait disturbances.

6) **Miscellaneous**

Example	**Effective in Treating**	**Side Effects**	**Nursing Implications**
L-asparaginase (an enzyme) (L-Asp, Elspar)	ALL (remission consolidation)	N&V, fever, azotemia, blood dyscrasias, diabetes, convulsions, personality changes, allergic reactions, anaphylaxis, reversible hepatotoxicity, pancreatitis	• Be alert to personality changes, including depression. • Monitor for signs of anaphylactic shock; have emergency equipment ready; consider skin-test results before giving dose. • Give antiemetics PRN. • Observe serum amylase levels periodically during therapy to detect pancreatitis.

Recommended References

"Fluids & Electrolytes." *NCP Guides #3:48, 49*, 2nd Ed., Nurseco, 1983.

"Leukemia: The Treatment of Leukemia," by A. Feeley & M. Houlihan. *Cancer Nursing*, June 1981:233–245.

The Nurse's Drug Handbook, 2nd Ed., by S. Loeble et al. New York: Wiley, 1980.

"The Patient with Leukemia." *NCP Guide #4:13*, 2nd Ed., Nurseco, 1983.

Physicians' Desk Reference, 36th Ed. Oradell, NJ: Medical Economics, 1982.

Practical Cancer Chemotherapy, by S. Rosenthal et al. Garden City, NY: Medical Examination Publishing, 1981.

Drugs: Antituberculous

GOAL: To reduce and control pathological changes and symptoms caused by tuberculosis infection; to stop the growth of tubercle bacilli; to render the Class III Tb patient noninfectious; to prevent Tb infection in the Class II patient (positive skin test, no other signs of disease).

General Considerations:

- **Dosage** of antituberculous drugs is based on body weight (approximately 10–25 mg/kg); all are administered orally except Streptomycin (SM) and Capreomycin (Capastat), which are given deep IM.
- **Excretion** of antituberculous drugs is mainly by the kidneys, therefore fluid intake and kidney function must be optimal.
- **Toxic effects** of these drugs often take place in the liver, so reduced dosages or alternative drugs must be used in those patients with poor liver function.
- Studies of *baseline* blood, liver, and renal function should be performed on all patients before chemotherapy is started. Normally these include WBC, hematocrit, platelet count, BUN, SGOT, bilirubin, and urinalysis. If the patient is sensitive or resistant to the primary drugs of choice, susceptibility studies will be done to determine proper alternative drugs.
- **Sputum examinations** are done monthly until sputum converts to nontransmitter status, then the sputum is examined every two months for the remainder of therapy, which must last at least six months after the sputum converts to negative.
- Anti-Tb drugs are given in combinations of two or more, daily or biweekly, for at least nine months; they are given longer to patients with extrapulmonary Tb or Tb complicated with another medical condition. Class II patients receive isoniazid (INH) for at least one year.
- **Current primary drugs of choice** are two bacteriocidal agents specific for mycobacterium tuberculosis: rifampin (Rifadin, Rimactane) and isoniazid (INH, Niconyl). Ethambutol (EMB, Myambutol), a bacteriostatic drug, may also be given. Combination drug products such as Mynah (ethambutol and isoniazid) and Rifamate or Rifanah (rifampin and isoniazid) have the advantage of reducing the number of pills an adult patient has to take. In children and elderly patients, dosage must be more individually adjusted.
- **Secondary drugs** are employed when there is drug resistance or poor tolerance to the primary drug choices. Streptomycin or Capreomycin are used when controlled therapy is necessary (with uncooperative or unreliable patients) or when the disease is extensive. Pyrazinamide (PZA), bacteriocidal especially against intracellular organisms, is useful to treat meningeal tuberculosis. Other drugs include ethionamide (ETHA, Trecator-SC, cycloserine [Seromycin], and prothinamide [Tremintrix]).

— **Nursing responsibilities** include obtaining and reinforcing firm commitment to complete long-term chemotherapy; instructing patient and family regarding side effects and adverse reactions to be noted and reported; observing for drug reactions, hypersensitivities, or unresponsiveness to chemotherapy; performing suitable monitoring tests for vision and hearing; obtaining blood and urine specimens for lab testing; and reporting and reviewing results with physician.

Drug	Side and Toxic Effects	Nursing Implications
isoniazid (INH, Niconyl, Nydrazid)	Optic & peripheral neuritis, hypersensitivity, hepatitis, convulsions	• Instruct pt. to report loss of appetite, nausea, vomiting, abdominal pain, dark urine, yellow skin or eyeballs, fatigue, malaise, weight loss, fever, aches in muscles or joints, skin rashes or itching; know that INH-related hepatitis occurs in less than 3% of pts., but risk increases with age or history of alcoholism; give pt. a written list of symptoms to note. • SGOT, SGPT may be ordered (a mild, self-limiting elevation may occur in 10% of pts.). • Pyridoxine (Vit. B 6) may be given concomitantly to prevent peripheral neuritis. • Keep monthly weight record.
rifampin (Rifadin, Rimactane, RIF)	Liver dysfunction, GI upset, thrombocytopenia, "flu-like" symptoms (myalgia, arthralgia, headache, fever), dyspnea, shock, renal failure, drowsiness	• Give on an empty stomach (a single dose before breakfast) to promote absorption & higher blood levels. • Monitor lab work & report abnormal values. • Observe for flu symptoms. • Warn pts. that medicine is reddish-brown & may color their urine, sputum, tears, other body secretions. • Increases liver breakdown (accelerates metabolism) of some drugs (steroids, warfarin, digoxin, oral hypoglycemics); monitor & report all untoward symptoms carefully so drug dosages may be adjusted.

Drug	Side and Toxic Effects	Nursing Implications
		• Warn pt. on oral contraceptives to take additional precautions, because pregnancy can occur. • Teach pt. that side & toxic effects are more likely to occur with sporadic rather than regular dosage, so avoid missing medication doses.
ethambutol (EMB, Myambutol)	Optic neuritis, skin rashes, GI tract irritation, hepatotoxicity, postural hypotension	• Assess baseline status of color perception (especially red & green) & visual acuity; observe vision changes & report promptly; perform Snellen eye chart exam and color-discrimination test monthly; examine skin monthly. • Question pt. regarding lightheadedness or dizziness when rising from a lying position. • Give medicine with or after meals.
streptomycin (SM)	Optic and vestibular toxicity, decreased hearing, vertigo, tinnitus, dermatitis	• Administer deep IM to minimize pain & irritation. • Observe pts., especially older ones, for adequate intake & output, hearing changes, ringing in ears (a forewarning sign), & rashes during each monthly check.
para-aminosalcylic acid (PAS)	GI tract irritation, anorexia, nausea, vomiting, diarrhea; skin rash; sodium loading; hepatotoxicity; gradual rise in body temp (102°–104°F.) in previously afebrile pts.	• Give with or after meals; may give with aluminum hydroxide gel; caution pt. against taking soda bicarb (a common practice) for any upset stomach. • Urge limitation of sodium, especially for elderly or overweight pts. with associated cardiac or renal disease. • Check & record temp each monthly visit; have pt. or family call in any elevation. • Check skin for rashes.
pyrazinamide (PZA, Zinamide)	Liver dysfunction, gout attacks	• Monitor liver function tests; observe & report gout symptoms so drugs to reduce hyperuricemia can be prescribed.

Recommended References

"Antitubercular Drugs have Unique Effects on Valium's Metabolism." *Nursing Drug Alert*, November 1981:103.

"Infectiousness of Pulmonary Tuberculosis after Starting Chemotherapy: Review of Available Data on an Unresolved Question," by R. Noble. *American Journal of Infection Control*, February 1981:2-6.

"Myambutol Can Precipitate Gouty Arthritis." *Nursing Drug Alert*, June 1981:53.

"The Patient with Tuberculosis." *NCP Guide #4:16*, 2nd Ed., Nurseco, 1983.

"Rifampin Allergic Failure." *Nursing Drug Alert*, January 1981:5-6.

"Short-course Chemotherapy for TB," by J. Brody. *Patient Care*, January 30, 1981:107-124.

"Shortest Possible Acceptable, Effective Ambulatory Chemotherapy in Pulmonary Tuberculosis: Preliminary Report I," by M. Mehrotra et al. *American Review of Respiratory Diseases*, September 1981:239-244.

"TB or not TB?" by S. Hopkins. *Nursing Mirror*, July 29, 1981:32-33.

"There's a Greater Chance for Permanent TB Cure with Short Term Drug Therapy," by D. Pritzker. *American Lung Association Bulletin*, April 1981:2-7.

Evidence Collection: Rape/Sexual Assault

LONG TERM GOAL: Evidence of rape/sexual assault will be collected correctly and carefully so that it will be admissible in court.

General Considerations:

— **Evidence collection** is essential for successful prosecution of rape/sexual assault cases. Because physical evidence is objective and less subject to bias than testimony, it is powerful and persuasive in court. (Even though a victim may be undecided to prosecute or not, evidence is usually collected since this *initial visit is the only time* collection may be done.)

— **Types of evidence:** (1) *Physical*, includes the victim's clothes, blood or secretions on skin, scrapings from fingernails, foreign materials (gravel, threads, loose hair), and swabs (vaginal, anal, oral); (2) *medical record* documentation of findings.

— Evidence collection is done by a doctor and nurse during assessment and physical examination. Familiarize yourself with agency protocol for this procedure and follow it exactly.

— When you receive specimens of physical evidence, label them immediately and keep all evidence in sight until handed over to a law enforcement officer. This "*continuity of command*" is vitally important in order for the evidence to "hold up" in court. (If the evidence is left alone in a room, handed to another person, left on a desk, etc., a possibility exists for someone to tamper with it and it will be thrown out of court.)

— Be aware that you may be called to court to testify; usually this is just to verify your evidence collection and your charting of the victim's physical and emotional status. If you are asked to testify, call the investigator on the case who can help you prepare as to type of questions asked, etc. Many nurses' associations provide legal assistance as part of membership; if you are a member, contact them at this time.

— **Nursing responsibilities** include:

1) observing, examining, and charting victim's emotional and physical status;
2) *very* carefully collecting, handling, and labeling evidence, assuring that it stays within own possession until handed to law enforcement officer; and
3) being willing to appear in court if called upon to do so.

Specific Considerations, Potential Patient Outcomes, and Nursing Actions:

1) Collection of Physical Evidence	Evidence will be collected according to agency protocol in a manner that is legally admissible in court: — explain all procedures carefully to victim before they are carried out (this gives victim a degree of control & a feeling of safety);

- examination & collection should be done carefully & sensitively; forcing the victim in any way may only make her feel she is being raped again;
- refrain from interviewing during the pelvic exam & collection process, since the physical position is reminiscent of the rape/assault and her powerlessness; ensure that she is adequately draped & that a *warm* speculum is used;
- develop a collection routine that you follow *every* time, so that you will be able to verify your procedure if called upon to do so in court;
- perform the examination & collection carefully & accurately; label each specimen immediately when you receive it; do not rely on your memory to recall where specimen originated, etc.;
- scrape caked blood/secretions into a test tube or sterile container & label as to site; save any foreign materials in a container & label as to site;
- place all clothing in a *paper* bag, never in a plastic bag because moisture may accumulate causing a mold to grow on any secretions on the clothing, thus making this evidence unusable; if clothes are damp, air-dry them before bagging;
- keep all evidence in your possession only until you hand it over to law enforcement officer;
- after evidence collection is completed, provide victim with an opportunity to wash/cleanse/bathe PRN, & change clothes.

2) Recording Details

The patient's chart will reflect an objective, accurate, and detailed account of the pertinent data needed:

- describe immediate emotional/physical status of victim *upon arrival* in your presence;
- ask & record only what you need to know, e.g., *information that is relevant to victim's care & legal evidence*;
- note accurately statements of victim & witnesses (if any) since your memory may later be clouded or blocked;
- be sure to sign all statements made by you; include full names of other medical assistants or law officers present.

Recommended References

"The Patient Experiencing Powerlessness." *NCP Guide #5:34*, Nurseco, 1981.
"The Patient Experiencing Shame/Embarrassment." *NCP Guide #5:35*, Nurseco, 1981.

Physical Assessment—Part A: General Principles

Definition: The use of all senses (touch, smell, visualization, hearing) to determine the physical status of an individual.

GOAL: The patient's problems, nursing diagnoses, and care will be based in part on the findings of the immediate and ongoing physical assessment of the individual.

General Considerations:

— The **purpose** of the initial physical assessment is to provide baseline data on the physical status of the patient and to verify information obtained from the nursing history; subsequent assessments identify changes from the baseline data.

— **Proficiency** in physical assessment comes with knowledge and practice of the essential skills. Knowledge can be acquired from books and peers, but skill comes only with practice, initially supervised and validated by someone with expertise.

— Physical assessment includes the **four basic techniques** of *inspection*, *palpation*, *percussion*, and *auscultation*; refer to the next three NCP Guides for specific information on each.

— A **specific order of assessment** is followed: it is a *head-to-toe sequence* that uses all four basic techniques for each body part before moving on to the next body part (some techniques will be eliminated as appropriate, e.g., the head is not percussed). The *area of pain or complaint* is examined *last* so that a thorough examination can be completed before the patient responds with anxiety to the favored area.

— **Instruments** used to enhance the senses are thermometer, flashlight, otoscope, ophthalmascope, stethoscope, BP cuff, tuning fork, tongue depressor, tape measure, and percussion hammer.

— **Physical assessment findings:** the nurse reports the patient's status by describing the physiological change (not the medical diagnosis) occurring in the body systems, e.g., inadequate pulmonary ventilation, alteration in level of consciousness, decreased body temperature.

— **Nursing responsibilities** include reviewing anatomy and physiology PRN (knowledge of anatomy is essential to accurate performance of physical assessment and knowledge of physiology is essential to accurate evaluation of findings); obtaining and recording physical data; relating the findings to the patient's history, chief complaint, and review of systems (subjective data); planning nursing care based on the current physical status; and evaluating physical responses to treatment.

Specific Considerations and Nursing Actions:

1) Psychologic Preparation	Provide simple descriptions for all assessment procedures before each is carried out; give slow, clear directions as to what you expect the patient to do; do not assume the patient can read your mind or "just know" what to do.

2) Environmental Management	Provide warm room; drape patient properly and adequately; use clean instruments; use sufficient light to visualize body parts and patient responses.
3) Body Changes and Chronic Health Problems	Pay specific attention to body changes related by the patient during the history; e.g., the patient states s/he had a broken leg at 14; examine the leg for scarring, mobility, color, & any other possible residual effects; assess patient based on family history of specific diseases, e.g., hypertension, diabetes, cancer. Assess for changes associated with risk factors; e.g., smoking, obesity, malnutrition, alcohol, and drug use.
4) Body Position	This facilitates examination and varies with part being assessed. The general rules are:

Position	**Body Area to be Assessed**
Seated on edge of bed, knees bent	Head, eyes, ears, nose, mouth, and neck. Shoulders, arms, hands, and fingers. Lungs, heart, lymph nodes, spinal column, knees, neural exam of face, upper extremities and reflexes, vital signs.
Lying flat	Breasts, lungs, heart, abdomen, groin, peripheral pulses, ROM, genitalia.
Standing	Posture, lower extremities, gait, spinal column, breasts, skin.

5) Evaluation and Recording of Findings	Evaluate all findings according to expected norms and developmental status of the individual; refer to NCPGs #3:22-26, "Normal Growth and Development," & #2:33, "Physiology of Aging." Report and chart findings; include all data gathered via the four basic assessment techniques; refer to NCPGs #4:48-50 for examples of recording of findings (both normal & deviations). Prescribe nursing care based on physical assessment findings. Evaluate care given based on patient's physical response, subjective data, and expected outcomes.

Recommended References

"Charting: Document Your Care Daily and Fully," by E. Eggland. *Nursing 80*, February 1980:38-44.
Clinical Manual of Health Assessment by J. Thompson and A. Bowers. St. Louis: Mosby, 1980.
"False Alarms in Assessing the Aged," by A. Tichy et al. *RN*, September 1981:58-62.
A Guide to Physical Examination, 2nd Ed., by B. Bates. Philadelphia: Lippincott, 1979.
Health Assessment, 2nd Ed., by L. Malasanos et al. St. Louis: Mosby, 1981.
"Patient Assessment—Based on Data, Not Intuition," by M.J. Mallick. *Nursing Outlook*, October 1981:600-604.
"Physical Assessment—Parts B: Inspection; C: Palpation and Percussion; and D: Auscultation." *NCP Guides #4:48-50*, 2nd Ed., Nurseco, 1983.
"Teaching Assessment of Client Functioning," by M. Jacoby and D. Adams. *Nursing Outlook*, April 1981:248-250.

Physical Assessment—Part B: Inspection

Definition: The use of the sense of vision to gather information on each body part.

GOAL: To identify the normal characteristics and deviations of the body.

General Considerations:

— **Inspection involves** a *general observation* of the patient's body movements for coordination and voluntary movement of skeletal muscles and an inspection of each body part.

— **Nursing responsibilities** include carrying out a general observation of the body from head to toe, and inspecting each body part, relating the findings to the patient's distress, and recording the findings in terms of what was/was not observed.

General Observation: record your findings in a manner descriptive enough to provide the reader with an overall picture of the patient.

Example:

Ms. R. is a 5' 7", 150-pound Hawaiian female with green eyes and shoulder-length brown hair. Her hair shines and is combed; nails are manicured and polished. She is wearing a blue blouse, navy-blue suit, and pink lipstick. On approaching her, she makes eye contact, uses a firm handshake, smiles and responds to the introduction with her name. She sits upright in the chair with feet flat on the floor and hands folded in her lap, head erect. She is able to state the reasons for her visit and freely asks questions when she wants to know something. She is not in distress and there are no visible deformities.

Specific Area of Inspection	Examples of Findings
Skin—note	
• *color*, *edema*, *lesions*, and *condition* of nails. Identify color in general and any deviation, including flushing, jaundice, cyanosis, or pallor.	"Skin color beige; cheeks flushed; nail beds pink; no edema noted"
Skin lesion classification	
• *primary* lesions are those that emerge from intact skin. These include:	"Brown macules intermittently across upper and lower extremities"
1) circumscribed, flat, nonpalpable changes in skin color (e.g., macule, patch)	"2 cm ulcer on calf of right lower extremity"

Specific Area of Inspection	**Examples of Findings**
Skin lesion classification	
2) palpable, elevated masses (e.g., tumor, wheal)	
3) circumscribed, superficial elevations, formed by free fluid in a cavity within the skin layers (e.g., vesicle, pustule)	
• *secondary* lesions are those that result from a change in the primary lesion. These include crusts, scales, excoriation, fissures, scars, and striae.	"Several white scales and reddened area over both elbows" "5 cm diagonal scar in left lower quadrant of abdomen"
• *vascular* lesions are those that occur in the vasculature and include cherry angiomas, spider angiomas, and venous stars.	"1 mm round, brownish cherry angiomas noted over hands and arms"
• *purpuric* lesions are those that occur in response to bleeding and include petechia and ecchymosis.	"Irregular 3 cm purplish area of ecchymosis noted on right foot"
Head—inspect	
• *hair* for color, quantity, distribution, cleanliness, length, texture	"Hair brown, thick, coarse, shoulder-length, evenly distributed, clean & shiny;
• *scalp* for presence/absence of lesions, scales	scalp clear; no dandruff or lesions noted;
• *face and skull* for symmetry, lesions, color, and contour.	face & skull symmetrical, beige skin, square shaped, no lesions noted"
Eyes—inspect	
• *sclera* for color	"Sclera white;
• *pupils* for equality, shape, symmetry, reflexes,and reaction to light	pupils equally round; both react & accommodate to light;
• *conjunctiva* for condition and color	conjunctiva pink, glistening;
• *total area* for symmetry, discharge, opacity, tearing	eyes symmetrical, no discharge or opacity noted; tearing elicited;
• *movement of eyelids*	freely movable eyelids; no ptosis or excessive blinking"

Specific Area of Inspection	Examples of Findings
Ears—inspect	
• *canals* for discharge • *external area* for lesions • *both ears* for symmetry	"Yellow discharge both ears; red, 2 cm patch noted over back lobe, left ear; ears symmetrical"
Nose—inspect	
• *internal nostrils* for patency, discharge • *mucous membranes* for color and condition • test *sense of smell* with alcohol or coffee	"Nostrils patent, no discharge noted; mucosa pink & glistening; sense of smell intact for alcohol/coffee"
Mouth—inspect	
• *lips and mucosa* for color and condition • *teeth* for number and condition • *tonsils* for absence/presence and condition • *gag reflex* for presence/absence • *gums, hard and soft palate* for condition • *speech* for pace, clarity, vocabulary, tone, and strength of voice	"Lips pink, moist, & smooth; all upper & lower teeth present, molars gold-capped; tonsils absent; gag reflex present; gums pink, no evidence of bleeding; palate pink, glistening, no lesions noted; slow, slurred, hoarse, soft voice; uses simple words & sentences"
Neck—inspect	
• *movement* • *distention* • *observable pulsations* or *enlarged thyroid* • *position of trachea*	"Freely movable; no distention noted; venous pulsation noted on left side; no enlargement of thyroid; trachea in midline"
Chest and Back—inspect	
• *respiratory movement*, both inhalation and exhalation • *shape of chest* • *spinal alignment* • *size, shape, and symmetry of breasts*	"Inhalation deep, exhalation shallow; chest concave; normal curvature of spine; breasts large, round; right breast slightly larger than left"

Specific Area of Inspection	Examples of Findings
Abdomen—inspect	
• *shape, size, fat distribution*	"Round, protuberant; fat distributed over entire area"
Extremities—inspect	
• type of *gait*	"Wide-based gait;
• *range of motion* during normal activity	able to move all extremities without assistance;
• *posture*	posture erect, no stooping noted;
• *hands, fingers, feet, & toes* for size, shape, mobility, reaction to stimuli	all fingers & toes noted, freely movable; no edema or clubbing noted; react to painful stimuli"
Genitalia and Rectal Area—inspect	
• *development*	"External genitalia present & fully developed; vaginal
• *mucous membranes* for color and condition	opening observed; mucous membrane pink & glistening;
• *hair* for color and distribution	brown hair distributed over genital region;
• *rectal area* for condition	no hemorrhoids observed; rectal opening intact"

Recommended References

"Common Skin Changes in the Elderly," by D. Uhler. *American Journal of Nursing*, August 1978:1342–1344.
"Examining the External Eye," by H. Boyd-Monk. Part I, *Nursing 80*, May 1980:58-63. Part II, Nursing 80, June 1980:58-63.
"Examining the Nose," by J. Malkiewicz. *RN*, April 1982:55–57.
"How to Assess the Ears and Test Hearing Acuity," by J. Malkiewicz. *RN*, March 1982:56–63.
"The Integumentary System," by J. Malkiewicz. *RN*, December 1982:55–60.
"Oral Assessment: How to Do It," by J. Schweiger et al. *American Journal of Nursing*, April 1980:654–657.
"Patient Assessment: Examining Joints of the Upper and Lower Extremities." *American Journal of Nursing*, April 1981:763–785.
"A Pragmatic Approach to Musculoskeletal Assessment," by J. Malkiewicz. *RN*, November 1982:57–62.
"Screening for Skin Cancer," by L. Schulmeister. *Nursing 81*, October 1981:42–45.
"Taking a Close Look at the Eye," by R. King. *RN*, February 1982:49–56.
"Tattletale Lesions," by T. Rosen and J. Mills. *RN*, September 1981:42–43.
"What Assessing the Mouth Can Tell You," by J. Malkiewicz. *RN*, May 1982:65–69.

Physical Assessment—Part C: Palpation and Percussion

Definition: The use of the sense of touch to determine the physical status of a body organ or part.

GOAL: To identify the normal characteristics, areas of tenderness and deviation, and vibratory response of the body.

General Considerations:

— **Palpation** is a technique that uses the sense of touch to distinguish the following variations in response: rough or smooth; hard or soft; stillness or vibration; heat or cold; and to feel for tissue changes such as tumors. It is performed by utilizing the fingers and hands according to areas of sensitivity; in general, finger tips are most sensitive to touch, palm and lateral aspect of hand are most sensitive to vibration, and dorsum (back) of hand is most sensitive to temperature.

— **Percussion** is the striking of a portion of the body to produce a shock wave that results in vibration. The vibration produces sound waves that can be interpreted as various types of sounds.

- *Technique:* place middle finger of one hand flat and firm against the area to be percussed. With the tip of the middle finger of the other hand, strike the distal joint of the middle finger that is flat and firm.
- *Areas to be percussed* include the interspaces of the anterior and posterior chest, the liver, the diaphragm, and the abdomen.
- *The significance of the findings* is related to the sound response elicited. Specific areas of the body have specific, normal sound responses that reflect the density of the tissue being percussed:

	Example
— *flatness* reflects a predominance of solid tissue in the body part	sound elicited over thigh
— *dullness* reflects more solid tissue than air in body part	sound elicited over liver
— *resonance* reflects more air than solid tissue in body part	sound elicited over normal lung
— *tympany* reflects a predominance of air in a body part	sound elicited with gastric air bubble or puffed-out cheek; largest amount of air is found in the intestine.

- **Abnormal responses** occur when the normal sound response is replaced by another type of sound. Remember, the sound produced reflects the density of the tissue being percussed. The density of the area is related to the amount of air, fluid, or solid tissue contained within it: e.g., dullness replaces resonance over the lungs when there is fluid or solid tissue in the lung or pleural space.

— **Nursing responsibilities** include determining the need and extent of palpation and percussion to be performed, reporting and charting findings (both normal and deviations) so that others are aware of the extent of the examination, and evaluating the significance of the findings in relation to the rest of the physical assessment and the physical status of the patient. All recording of findings should include areas palpated and percussed and body response to the assessment, e.g., breast palpation: breasts are symmetrical; no tenderness, lesions, discharge, dimpling, or skin retractions noted; no axillary or chest nodes palpable.

Specific Areas of Palpation and Percussion	**Examples of Findings**
Skin—note	
• *moisture, temperature, texture, edema, and turgor*. (Turgor is the assessment for skin elasticity. It is either present, diminished, or absent. Normal skin should return to pre-pinched state immediately after being pinched. Any lag would suggest diminished turgor.)	"Skin dry, warm to touch, smooth, no edema noted" "Turgor diminished and takes 5 sec (note number of seconds) to return to place"
Head—palpate	
• for *lesions, texture of hair, areas of tenderness, status of fontanels in infant*	"Tenderness noted in occipital area; hair coarse" "Anterior fontanel open"
Face—palpate	
• for *lesions, areas of tenderness*	"Papules present and evenly distributed over face; no areas of tenderness noted"
Eyes—palpate	
• for *condition* and *movement of eyelids*	"Eyelids freely movable; edema noted on eyelids"
Ears—palpate	
• for *mobility*	"Ears and nose freely movable"
Nose and Mouth—palpate	
• for *lesions*, *areas of tenderness*.	"Papule noted on inner, upper right side of mouth"

Specific Areas of Palpation and Percussion	Examples of Findings
Neck—palpate • for *enlarged nodes, location, and presence of thyroid gland, carotid artery, tracheal position, and movement of neck*	"No nodes palpable; thyroid palpable but not enlarged; carotid artery palpable but unequal in rate: left side = 80, right side = 72 (state rate); trachea midline, neck moves through full ROM"
Chest and Back—palpate • *nodes, respiratory rate and rhythm, breasts, axillary nodes, supra- and infraclavicular nodes* • *respiratory excursion* (the range and symmetry of finger movements noted during inhalation and exhalation on posterior chest: place thumbs at level of and parallel to 10th rib, hands slightly grasping rib cage; have thumbs slightly touching and just together, parallel at the spinal column. Ask patient to inhale deeply and watch the movement of the thumbs away from the midline. Lag or impairment of thoracic movement suggests underlying deviations from normal), percuss *interspaces* of anterior and posterior chest; expect resonance in all areas except over the heart (anterior chest)	"Respirations 20, even, deep; supraclavicular nodes palpable; hard, circumscribed, 2 cm lesion present in right breast at 1 o'clock; no discharge, tenderness, dimpling, nipple retraction, or asymmetry noted in breasts. Resonance noted on both sides over posterior back to level of diaphragm"
Abdomen—palpate and percuss • in *all quadrants* for edema, lesions, areas of tenderness, and vibratory response	"Large, soft abdomen with generalized tenderness noted; dullness heard over liver, otherwise tympany noted"
Extremities—palpate • *pulses* (femoral, posterior, tibial, popiteal, pedal) for rate, rhythm, and equality bilaterally • for *lesions*, *mobility*, areas of *tenderness*, response to stimuli	"Femoral, posterior, tibial, popiteal, & pedal pulses palpable and equal bilaterally; rate of 80; rhythm even. No lesions noted. Left side, arm, & leg unmovable without assistance; no response to painful stimuli. Right side within normal limits"

Specific Areas of Palpation and Percussion

Genitalia and Rectal Area—palpate

- for *lesion, tenderness, patency* of opening, *mobility* of male organs and foreskin, external *hemorrhoids.*

Examples of Findings

"Vaginal opening intact, mucosa pink, glistening & no lesions noted. Rectal opening intact; 2 1-cm hemorrhoids noted on left side of anal opening"

Recommended References

"Abdominal Assessment—A Blending of Science and Art," by C. Smith. *Nursing 81*, February 1981:42-49.

Assessing Your Patients, Nursing Photobook Series. Springhouse, PA: Intermed Communications, Inc., 1980.

"Detailed Guidelines for a Thorough Examination of the Heart," by R. King. *RN*, July 1982:57-63.

"Exploring the Neck and Lymphatics," by R. King. *RN*, June 1982:49-55.

"Physical Assessment—Part A: General Principles." *NCP Guide #4:47*, 2nd Ed., Nurseco, 1983.

"Physical Assessment—Part B: Inspection." *NCP Guide #4:48*, 2nd Ed., Nurseco, 1983.

"Your Fingers on the Pulse—Evaluating What You Feel," by C. Pepler. *Nursing 80*, November 1980:33-39.

Physical Assessment—Part D: Auscultation

Definition: The use of the sense of hearing to listen to the sounds produced by the human body.

GOAL: To identify normal, deviations from, and changes in body sounds.

General Considerations:

— **Auscultation** is done by means of an instrument to aid hearing, utilizing a stethoscope with a bell and diaphragm. The bell side is best for low-pitched sounds; the diaphragm side is best for high-pitched sounds. Successful auscultation means listening to only one sound at one time.

— **Body sounds** fall into two major categories: those produced by the *thoracic or abdominal organs or viscera* and those produced by the *movement of blood* in the cardiovascular system.

— Breath sounds are auscultated over the trachea, mainstem bronchus, and at the intercostal spaces on the anterior and posterior chest:

normal breath sounds include:

- *bronchial:* a tubular sound that is louder on expiration, heard over the area of the trachea
- *vesicular:* a sound resembling wind blowing through trees causing leaves to rustle; louder on inspiration, heard over peripheral lung
- *bronchovesicular:* heard over area of mainstem bronchus; resembles bronchial sounds on expiration and vesicular sounds on inspiration.

abnormal breath sounds include:

- *rales:* discrete, noncontinuous sounds produced by moisture in the tracheobronchial tree; not cleared by coughing; sound can be simulated by rolling a lock of hair near the ear
- *rhonchi and wheezes*: continuous sounds produced by air flow across passages narrowed by secretions, mucosal swelling, tumors:
  - — sibilant (high-pitched wheezing sound)
  - — sonorous (low-pitched, moaning, or snoring quality; coughing may alter sounds)
- *friction rubs*: cracking, grating sounds originating in an inflamed pleura; coughing has no effect on them
- *presence of breath sounds* in location other than where normally found.

— **Abdominal sounds** are auscultated over the total abdominal area according to quadrants. It is easiest to divide the abdominal region into four quadrants:

Right	1	3	Left
side	2	4	side

1 and 2 are considered the right upper and lower quadrants (RUQ,RLQ)
3 and 4 are considered the left upper and lower quadrants (LUQ,LLQ)

a) *bowel sounds* are the result of movement of air and fluid through the GI tract; they occur approximately every 5–15 seconds and sound like bubbles, gurgles, growls
b) *peristaltic sounds* reflect bowel muscle functioning and may be irregular. Listen for at least five minutes before determining that these sounds are absent; frequency is directly related to the status of the digestive process.

— **Cardiac sounds** are auscultated:
a) over the site of the carotid artery and thyroid
b) at four points on the chest wall that reflect where the sounds of the heart valves are best heard:
- *aortic area*: 2nd right intercostal space at the sternal border
- *pulmonic area*: 2nd left intercostal space at the sternal border
- *tricuspid area*: 5th left intercostal space at the sternal border
- *mitral (apical) area*: 5th left intercostal space just medial to the midclavicular line

c) to determine the nature of S_1 and S_2 (lub-dub)
- S_1 is the 1st heart sound (lub) and it reflects closure of the atrioventricular valves (mitral and tricuspid)
- S_2 is the 2nd heart sound (dub) and it reflects closure of the semilunar valves (aortic and pulmonic)

d) abnormal sounds are numerous and include physiological and pathological murmurs, split sounds, opening snap, ejection clicks, and an abnormal 3rd and 4th heart sound.

— **Nursing responsibilities** include being aware of landmarks on anterior and posterior chest, being skilled at identifying normal sounds of the chest and abdomen, understanding the relationship of sounds heard to the physical status of the patient, and reporting and charting findings according to location, quality, frequency, and intensity of sounds heard.

Specific Areas of Auscultation	Examples of Findings
Neck—auscultate	
• *carotid arteries* and area of thyroid	"Bruit noted in left carotid artery"
Chest and Back—auscultate	
• *breath sounds* at interspaces; cardiac sounds for S_1, S_2; listen for normal and note deviations	"Normal breath sounds, rales, rhonchi noted; click, gallop rhythm noted at mitral area"
Abdomen—auscultate	
• *abdominal sounds* in all quadrants; listen for one minute in each quadrant	"Constant bowel sounds heard in all quadrants"

Recommended References

"Abdominal Assessment—A Blending of Science and Art," by C. Smith. *Nursing 81*, February 1981:42-49.
"Assessing the Heart: What's Normal and What's Not," by J. Koeckeritz. *RN*, September 1982:59-63.
"Examining the Thorax and Respiratory System," by R. King. *RN*, August 1982:55-63.
"From Assessment to Intervention: How to Use Heart and Breath Sounds as Part of Your Nursing Care Plan," by B. Humbrecht and E. Van Parys. *Nursing 82*, April 1982:34-41.
"Hands-On Guide to Palpation and Auscultation," by C. Cannon. *RN*, March 1980:20-25.
"Honing your Respiratory Assessment Technique," by N. Blackburn and D. Cebenka. *RN*, May 1980:28-31.
"How to Hear it Right: Evaluating and Choosing a Stethoscope," by P. Stright and Sister M. Soukup. American *Journal of Nursing September 1977:1477.*
"Knowing What You Hear: A Guide to Assessing Breath and Heart Sounds," by M. Visich. Nursing 81, November 1981:64-76.
"Physical Assessment—Part A: General Principles." *NCP Guide #4:47*, 2nd Ed., Nurseco, 1983.
"A Simplified Introduction to Lung Sounds," by R. Murphy (a cassette). Wellesley, MA: Stethophonics, 1977.
"Systems and Signs: Respiration and Auscultation," by A. Roberts. *Nursing Times*, January 1981 (center supplement).
"What Those Breath Sounds are Telling You to Do," by B. Schare and C. Stehlin. *RN*, December 1981:55-63.